# THE
# ANTI AGEING
# FOOD &
# FITNESS
# PLAN
## PLANT BASED EDITION

BY RICK HAY **The SuperFoodist**

# Contributors

Fitness
Ian Chapman

Graphic Design
Robbie Mason

Additional Recipes and Recipe Photography
Daniela Fischer

Photography
Rick and Sarah Photos by Sean Smiles
Front and Back Cover Photos of Rick by Antonia Radich

Front Cover Design
Will Coddington

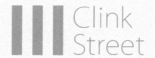

*Published by Clink Street Publishing*
*Copyright © 2019*

*First Edition 2019*

*ISBN: 978-1-913136-90-1*
*E-Book: 978-1-913136-91-8*

# In the Press

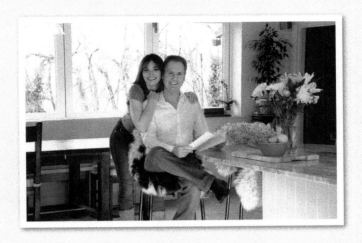

### The Daily Telegraph
'The Anti Ageing Food and Fitness Plan is specifically designed to counter age related weight gain by increasing metabolism'

### Fit and Well
'You can lose 2lb a week easily and sensibly with the eating plan from superfood expert Rick Hay'

### Bella
'The Anti Ageing Diet – lose up to 5lb in 7 days'

### Prima Magazine
'Feel Younger Fitter and Leaner'
'Drop a few years with this easy Anti Ageing Food and Fitness Plan'

### Healthista
A healthy twelve week transformation that delivers weight loss the easy way.

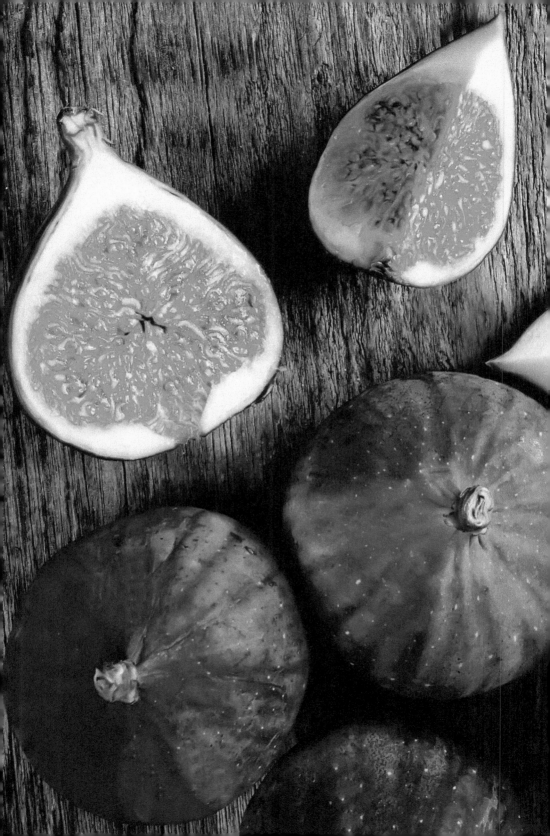

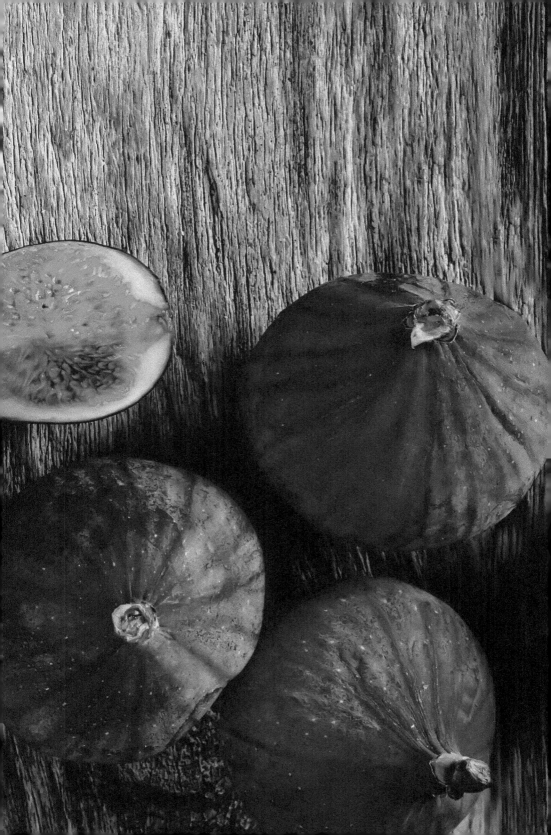

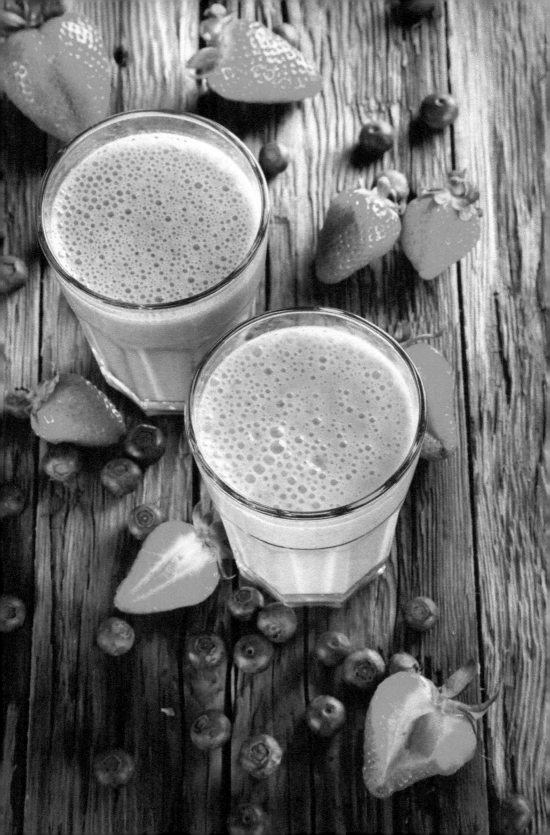

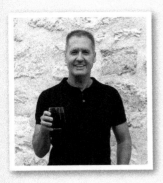

# Rick Hay

**The Superfoodist –
Dip Nutrition, Dip Botanical Medicine,
Dip Iridology, Dip Teaching**

Rick is an anti ageing and fitness nutritionist with many years clinical experience in nutrition, naturopathy, botanical medicine and iridology.

His specialisms include obesity treatment, weight management, anti-ageing nutraceuticals, beauty from within supplements and natural sports medicine options.

Rick lectures in Sustainable Weight Management and Detox at The College of Naturopathic Medicine in London and is a regular Health and Fitness Expert on Ideal World TV.

He is the Nutritional Director and Formulator at Healthista.
Rick's vast experience in Nutrition, Botanical Medicine and Nutraceutical Formulation has led to him being regularly sought after by the media both in the UK and Australia for his nutritional expertise and comment.

His approach is to debunk the myths and misinformation surrounding diets, healthy eating and weight management.
He is passionate about the science behind food and fitness and aims to provide easy, yet effective nutritional solutions.
He also has released three Vibrapower Fitness DVD's in conjunction with Ideal World TV and regularly features in many healthy eating and fitness videos.

Rick is an advocate of more plant based eating and follows a plant based diet himself.

For more information and inspiration go to www.rickhay.co.uk and www.healthista.com

# Sarah Parish

**British Film, TV and Theatre Actor**

With my hectic schedule I was finding it increasingly more difficult to stay in shape. I'd gone from a size 10 to a 12 / 14 in six months and I was exhausted. I knew if I kept going I'd have a middle aged figure – tummy spread, loose skin between the legs, cellulite – which also comes with the depression, the stress, the tiredness. I needed another way.

I was looking for something that would provide results that were achievable and sustainable - I wanted to get in shape the smart way. 'I was complaining to a health-conscious friend about not being able to shift fat at the sides of my thighs, stomach and around my back and she said, 'There's someone I want you to meet.' That's how I met Rick Hay, an Australian nutritional therapist who lectures in Sustainable Weight Management at London's College of Naturopathic Medicine.

When I talked to Rick and looked into the science behind both the healthy eating and fitness components of the plan I was really impressed. Fad diets or complicated exercise regimes are definitely not what I need. The nutritional philosophy really resonated with me - the plan delivers nutrient density, cellular health and anti ageing benefits with no calorie counting.

Rick also taught me about the importance of building muscle with HIIT training and eating enough healthy protein and nutrient rich foods to keep skin firm. Within eight weeks on my original plan I had dropped a dress size - and another soon followed.

I now include more plant based options in my diet as I am aware of the many health benefits that foods that are higher in fibre deliver beyond that just of weight loss. I also have incorporated some LISS workouts into my fitness regime.

**Sarah Parish**

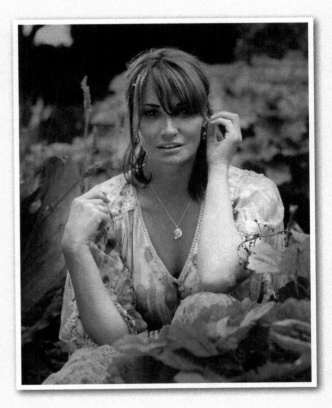

NB Sarah followed the original edition of 'The Anti Ageing Food and Fitness Plan' and incorporates many of the new plant based recipes featured in this new edition into her diet.

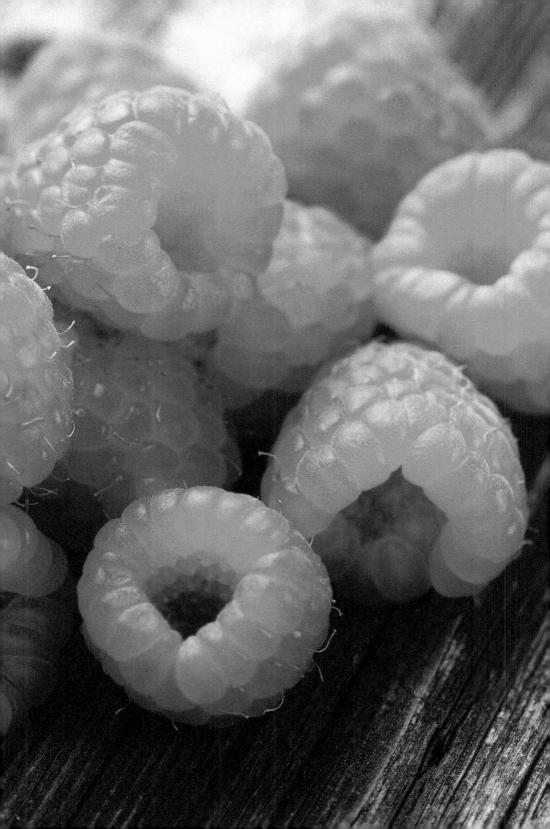

# CONTENTS

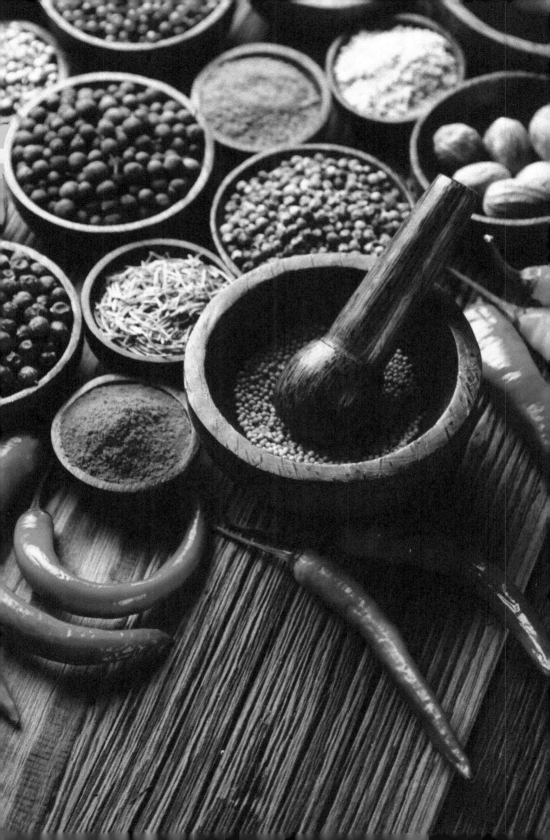

# INTRODUCTION

I have been writing and talking about the benefits of eating more plant based protein for all of my career so it came as no surprise that when a study by JAMA Internal Medicine looked at the diet data for 130,000 people they found that there was a reduced mortality rate in people who ate more plant based protein.

There was a higher mortality risk in those who ate more animal proteins and with just a 3% increase in calories from plant protein the risk of death was reduced by 10%.

In summary you can boost your life expectancy by eating more plant based protein vs animal protein.

With this in mind this new plant based plan targets ageing at a cellular level using nutrient dense meals, snacks and supplements. The fitness component combines both high intensity interval training with low intensity steady state exercise to deliver faster results. The plan has been designed to achieve the best anti ageing, fitness and weight loss outcomes over a 12 week period.

The selected foods, herbs and spices promote fat metabolism and improve digestive function whilst helping to control cravings and improve satiety. There are also benefits to heart health.

The meals and snacks provide low glycaemic load nutrient density to keep blood sugar levels steady and to boost both immunity and energy production.

The addition of plant based protein powders are recommended throughout the plan in order to increase the protein content of your smoothies.
This will help to keep you feeling fuller for longer, keep cravings at bay, improve concentration and increase energy levels.

You can continue the plan beyond the twelve week transformation period or you can tweak it to create your own version. It is ok to repeat four weeks of the plan at regular intervals throughout the year if you need to get back on track or have a special event coming up.

Including more plant based meals in your diet and moving more are integral to achieving an improvement in overall health.

# What's it all about?

Eating a diet that is made up of nutrient dense plant based protein has been shown to increase life expectancy whilst lowering the incidence of many of today's common disease states such as cardiovascular problems, diabetes and obesity related illnesses.

At a cellular level the nutrient dense meal and snack options that are included in this plan have been chosen to optimise cellular function and to provide your body with all of the vitamins, minerals, electrolytes, antioxidants and phytonutrients that are required in order to achieve optimal health.

Providing the body with the right fuel optimises the trillions of biochemical reactions that take place every minute inside your body.

Some of these nutrients help to lengthen and protect telomeres, which in turn leads to a longer life span.

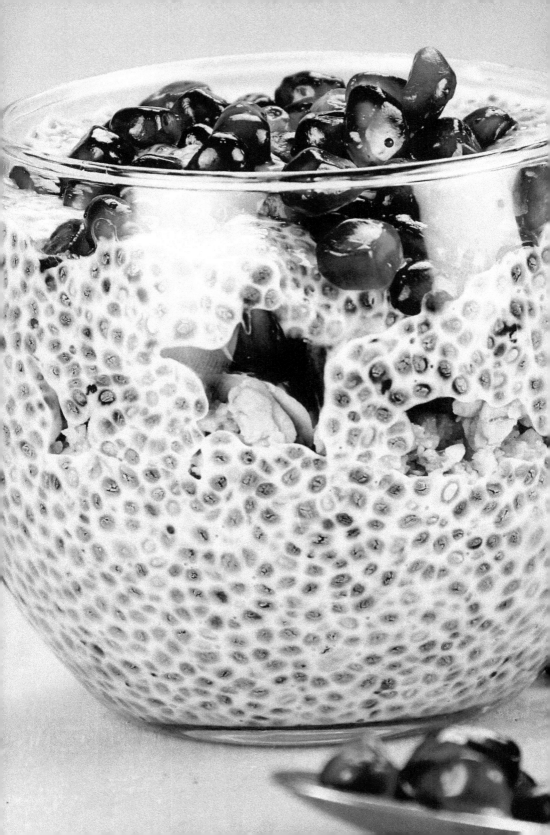

The food choices help with alkalisation and detoxification and will also help you to achieve correct digestive function – if your body is not eliminating correctly, the resulting toxic build up can speed up the ageing process and hamper any weight management campaign.

Spices are included in the plan as they are thermogenic and can have a positive effect on feelings of satiety and fat oxidisation. They also help to boost the immune system and have strong anti-inflammatory properties.

The consumption of these spices increases thermogenesis throughout the day and when combined with the intermittent fasting element of the plan may help to extend lifespan.

The first four weeks are all about a tune up - it is a time to eat more healthily and to move more. The plant based recipes deliver more fibre to the body which helps with the natural cleansing process and also helps with feelings of fullness.

Research is indicating that an increase in the consumption of plant based proteins helps with cardio vascular health.

Fibre rich fruits, vegetables and legumes provide an antioxidant and phytonutrient boost to help to support the immune system. Low GL recipes promote healthy digestive, immune, lymphatic and nervous system function.

The combination of HIIT (High Intensity Interval Training) and LISS (Low intensity Steady State) exercise will enhance this initial tune up period and increase physical performance. HIIT reduces telomere shortening which helps to slow down the ageing process whilst LISS helps with fat burning.

It is important that you stay hydrated whilst on the plan so make sure you are drinking enough filtered water especially when you are doing the exercise sections, or if you are doing the plan in the warmer months.

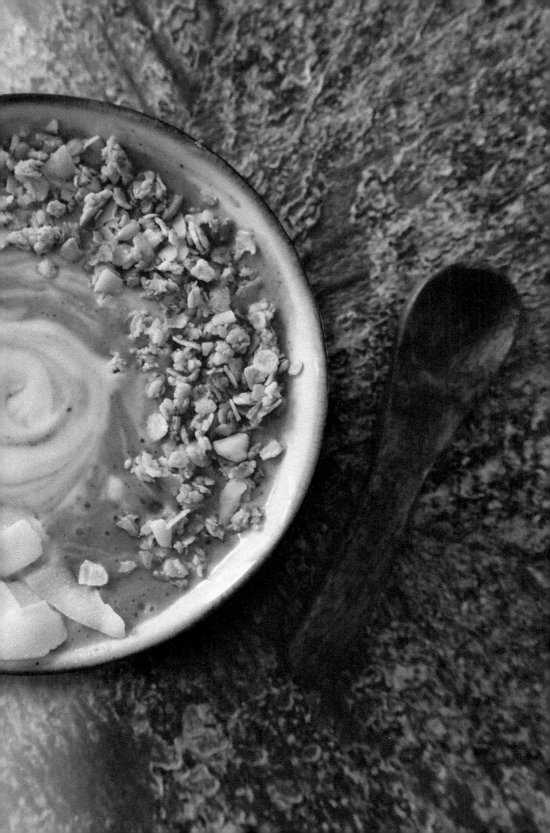

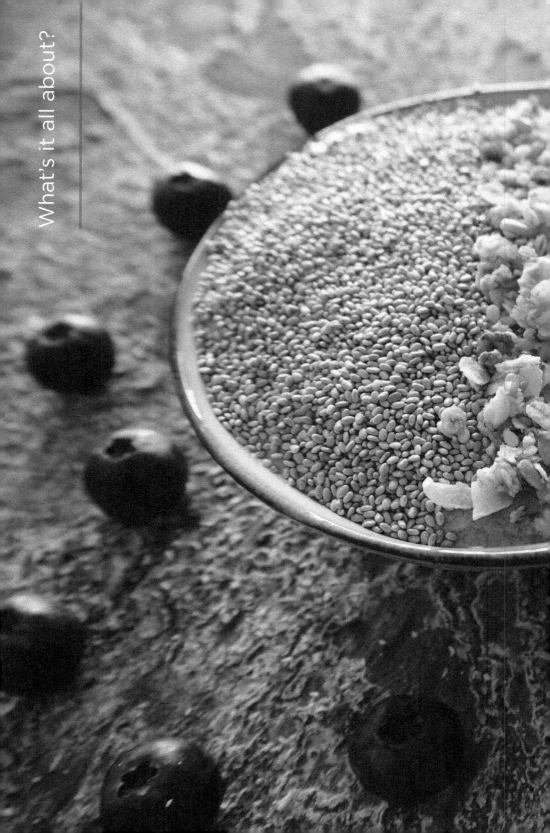

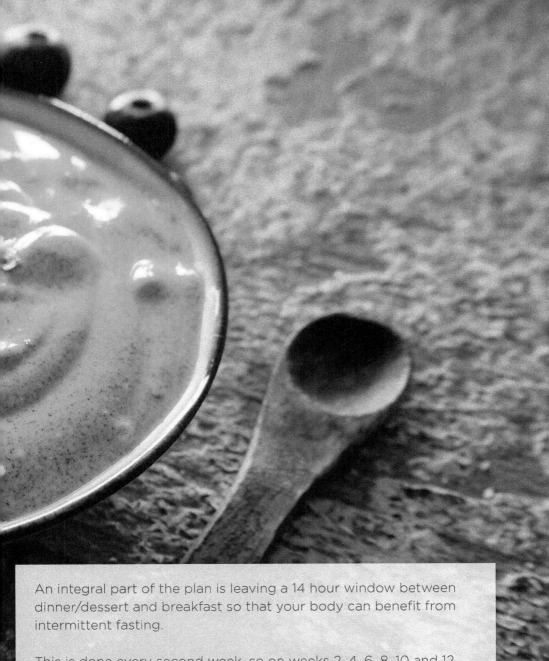

An integral part of the plan is leaving a 14 hour window between dinner/dessert and breakfast so that your body can benefit from intermittent fasting.

This is done every second week, so on weeks 2, 4, 6, 8, 10 and 12, you will need to have dinner a little earlier and breakfast a little later. When to do this is highlighted in the plan.

The Anti Ageing Food and Fitness Plan is not about counting calories but is focused on healthy food options that will deliver improved health outcomes whilst maintaining a healthy weight.

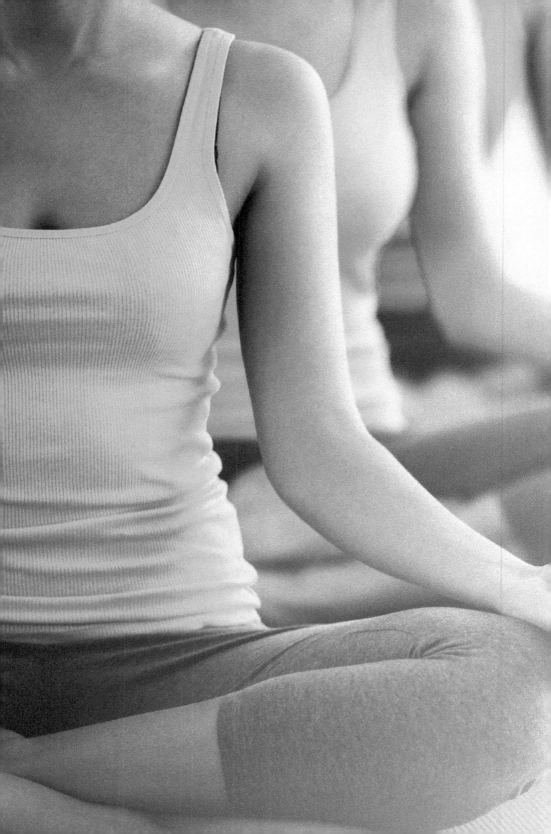

# Fitness Instructions

Exercise should form an integral part of any diet plan as movement is one of the best ways to slow down the ageing process. Research shows that even short bursts of exercise can help prevent and protect against an array of modern health issues.

Aim to implement movement and exercise into your daily routine and set approximately 3-4 times a week to do the specific exercise routines outlined in the Fitness Sections of your Anti Ageing Food and Fitness Plan.

The Cardio Circuit Challenges are based on the principle of HIIT – High Intensity Interval Training or Burst Training. HIIT is where intervals of low to moderate intensity training is alternated with short bursts of high intensity intervals.

This style of exercise creates a super charged cardio routine which enables you to burn fat at a faster rate and in less time. High Intensity Interval Training helps to speed up your metabolism and to burn more calories throughout the day – even after you finish exercising.

These exercises utilise your own body weight but if you wish to use some hand weights this will increase the resistance.

Low Intensity Steady State (LISS) exercises are also included. The combination of HIIT workouts when combined with some LISS exercise is an effective way to burn fat.

If you are a **Beginner** do each circuit once or twice giving you a total of 5-10 minutes of HIIT/Cardio.

If you are **Intermediate** do each circuit two or three times giving you a total of 10-15 minutes of HIIT/Cardio.

If you are **Advanced** do each circuit three or four times giving you a total of 15-20 minutes of HIIT/Cardio.

Rest for one minute between circuits.

### HIIT Weeks 1-4
Do each exercise in the circuit for 20 seconds intensely and then slowly for 40 seconds.
Each individual exercise within the circuit should be done for 1 minute.

### HIIT Week 5-8
Do each exercise in the circuit for 30 seconds intensely and then slowly for 30 seconds.
Each individual exercise within the circuit should be done for 1 minute.

### HIIT Weeks 9-12
Do each exercise in the circuit for 40 seconds intensely and then slowly for 20 seconds.
Each individual exercise within the circuit should be done for 1 minute.

Follow the 1 minute **Warm Up** routine before commencing each HIIT session, never work out cold muscles.
This will start to get the blood pumping and can assist by loosening up your joints.
It will also help to reduce the risk of injury.

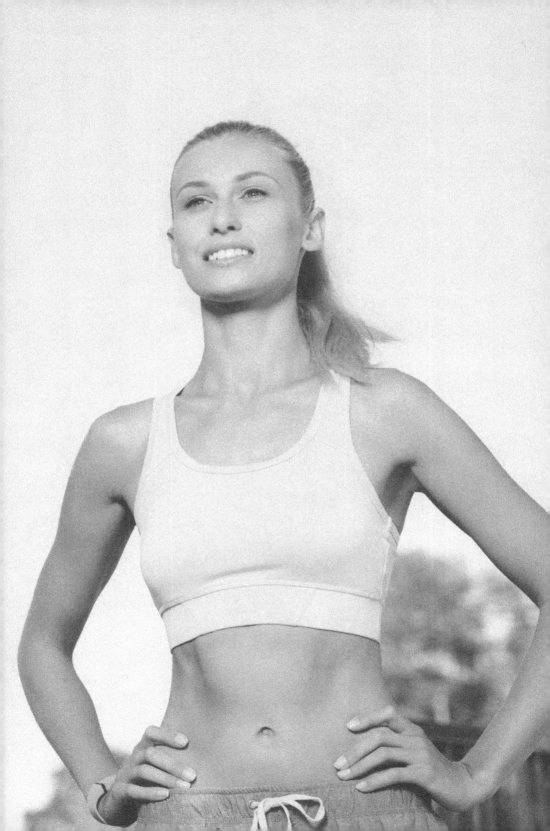

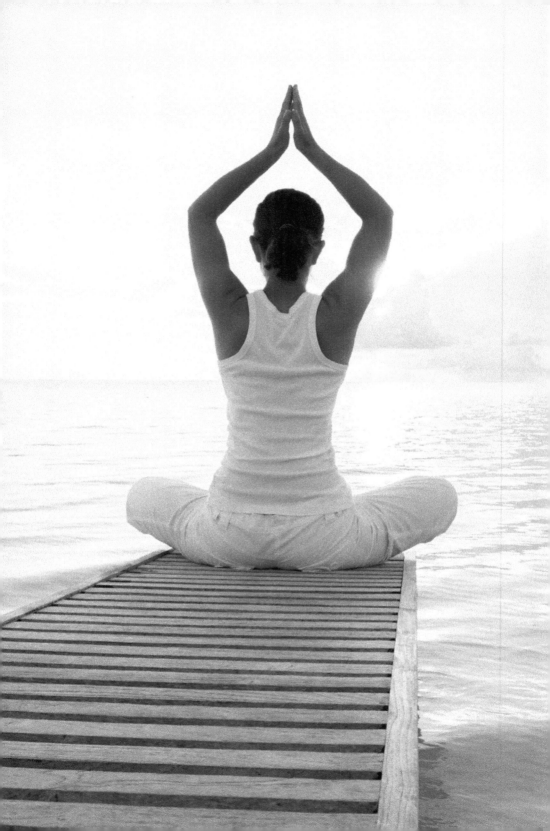

Included as well is a set of Yoga and Pilates type stretches designed to help you relax your muscles after the period of intense exercise. Always take at least 5 minutes or so after your HIIT session to perform these stretches – they will help to improve your flexibility and help to prevent soreness the next day.

To have an effective and successful exercise regime it is important to mix things up to add variety to your routine. Other activities will accelerate your results, such as playing a ball sport, swimming, cycling or jogging.

LISS - low intensity steady state - exercise helps to burn more fat too and may also help to decrease stress levels.

Another great idea is to use technology. One of the best examples of this is Vibration training. It consists of either a disc or a plate which produces a pivoting or oscillating motion much like that of a see-saw or trampoline. Exercising on a moving platform like this helps to work not only your core muscles but also your supporting stabilising muscles giving you a fuller body workout.

Incidental exercise can also really assist with weight management and fitness goals.
Try to walk more and to get the best results you can employ the principles of HIIT here as well – walk quickly for a minute then slower for 30 seconds and repeat.

It may also be a good idea to get a pedometer to count the number of steps that you are taking every day.

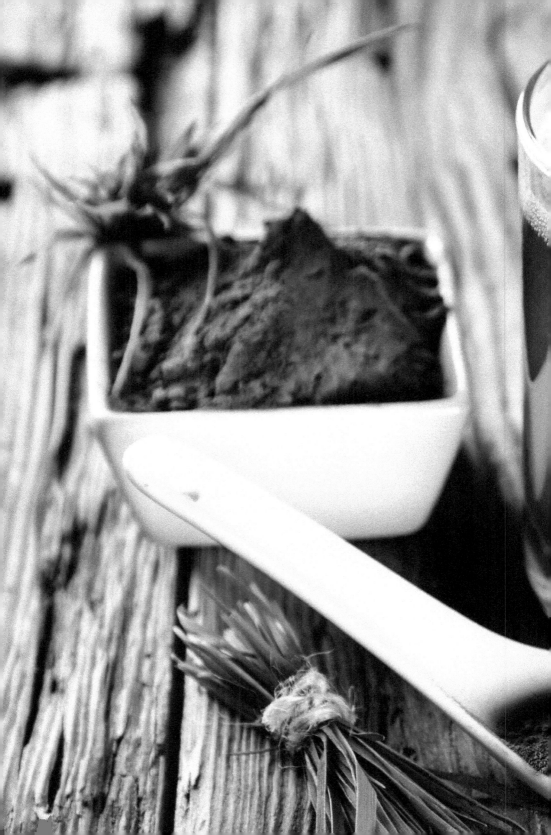

# Intro  Weeks 1 to 4

The first four weeks of the plan are all about introducing more high fibre plant based foods into your diet. These will help with the natural cleansing process and also delivers more colourful, antioxidant rich fruits and vegetables into the mix. There are three main meal nutrient dense, low glycaemic meal choices together with vitamin rich snack options and healthy, delicious desserts.

These will kick start your metabolism and reduce cravings and unhealthy snacking. The plan includes healthy carbohydrates to help with both cognition and energy levels. There is also the option to replace certain meals or snacks with plant based protein smoothies which can help to stimulate weight loss. They help to balance blood sugar levels which should result in more stable moods.

Unlike many fad diets no one food group is excluded - there is a combination of protein, carbohydrates and healthy fats.

The emphasis is on improving digestive health in order to optimise health outcomes. The recipes help with gut health – and with better digestive function comes improved liver function. You can expect better skin condition by the end of week two or three as a result.

It is also a time to look at removing chemical cleaning products that you may be using as these can result in endocrine disruption.
Anything that you are using for personal care from moisturisers to toothpastes should be natural and chemical free.

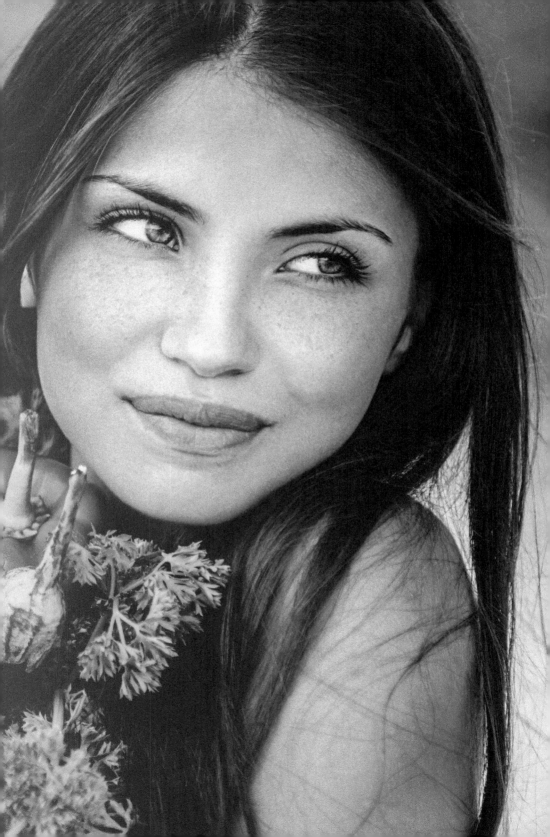

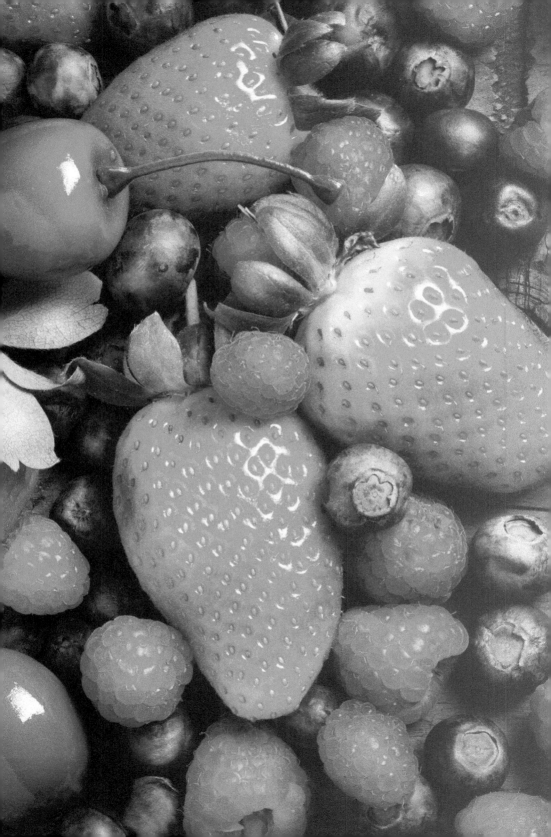

# Weeks
# 1&3

# Balance

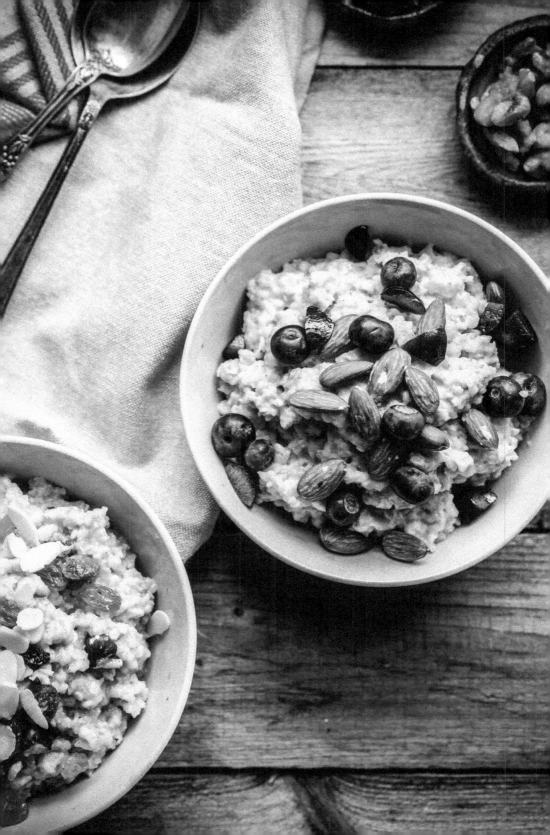

## Before Breakfast

### Lemon Blast

Half a glass of warm filtered water with the juice of half a lemon: to kick start the liver and gallbladder and digestive function. This is alkalising and helps with fat metabolism also.

# Breakfast

### Porridge with Berries

Add a few teaspoons of fresh or frozen berries to a small bowl of porridge.

Top with a dollop of coconut yogurt and a teaspoon of chia or sunflower seeds.

Berries are catabolic and help with fat burning and oats help to keep blood sugar levels stable which assist weight loss and mood.

### OR

### Avocado and Kale Protein Bowl

Blend • 1 cup kale leaves • 1 cup cashew milk • ½ banana • 1 scoop of plant based protein powder and ½ an avocado

Blend and transfer to bowl and add the following toppings: • 1 sliced kiwi • 1 tsp chia seeds and 1 tbsp goji berries

### OR

### Green Protein Smoothie

Blend 250 mls of rice or almond milk with 1 banana or with a cup of berries and a few almonds.

Add a handful of spinach or kale to increase green vegetable intake.

For extra protein add 1 scoop of plant based protein.

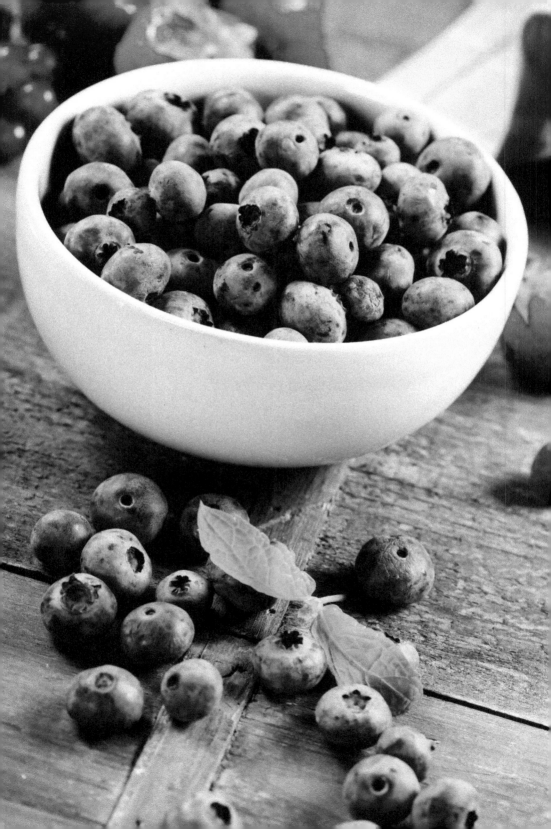

# Mid Morning

### Berry Bowl

To a small bowl of berries add a few almonds or cashews and a couple of teaspoons of coconut yogurt.

Eating every few hours helps to control portion size and helps to regulate blood sugar levels which should reduce cravings.

## OR

### Fruit with Almonds

1 apple or other piece of fruit, as desired, with a few almonds

## OR

### Coconut Yogurt

Small bowl of coconut yogurt together with half an apple or a few slices of melon

Have with one cup of fat burning matcha green tea or coffee.

Green tea or matcha green tea will stimulate fat burning and promote healthy circulation. Their bitter quality means that they are liver and gall bladder tonics.

Matcha green tea and green tea will also help to stimulate digestion in general.

Weight loss is more easily achieved if you have can stimulate sluggish digestion.

Do not sweeten with sugar or artificial sweeteners.

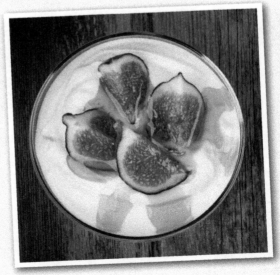

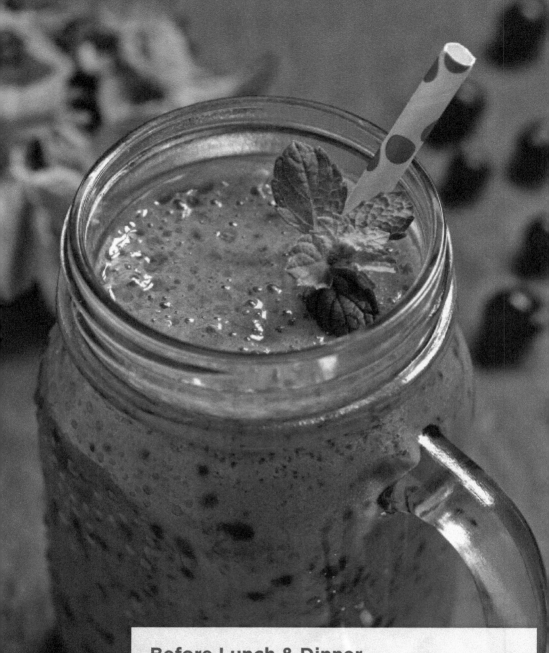

### Before Lunch & Dinner
**Spirulina Super Green Boost**
3 to 6 Spirulina or Super Green tablets can be taken as they help with feelings of fullness and with controlling portion size.
They also help to alkalise the system.

# Lunch

## Roasted Sweet Potato, Beans and Hummus Wrap

• ¼ sweet potato cubed • 2 tbsp hummus • 2 tbsp kidney beans • handful of spinach • teaspoon cumin • teaspoon turmeric • ¼ teaspoon black pepper • ¼ teaspoon salt • 1 tablespoon linseed oil

Preheat oven to 350°F.

Mix all the spices together and toss them over the sweet potatoes and beans.

Add 1 tablespoon of oil and toss them until the sweet potatoes are fully coated with the spices and oil.

Roast the mix for about 20-25 minutes until tender.

Remove from the oven to cool.

Spread 2 tablespoons of hummus on a wrap and add the ingredients and top it all with the fresh spinach.

## OR

## Lightly Fried Tofu or Tempeh

Lightly fry 150g or less of the tempeh or tofu in a little olive oil and serve with a cup of leafy greens.

Add an olive oil and balsamic vinegar dressing.

Season with thermogenic garlic, black pepper, turmeric, paprika or ginger.

This is a protein based meal that is high in antioxidants and delivers healthy omegas to help with mood and skin.

## OR

## Berry Smoothie

Blend • 250 mls of rice • hemp • coconut or almond milk with a cup of berries and a few slices of beetroot.

Add a 4 to 5 almonds or macadamias and/or 1 scoop of plant based protein to help with satiety and skin condition.

These shakes can be used as a meal replacement but only for one or two of the meals, not all three.

A half serve of the shake can also be used as mid morning or mid afternoon snack but not if it is being used as a meal replacement though.

## Mid Afternoon

### Nut Butter Corn Cake

Spread almond or cashew butter onto 1 or 2 vegan corn or rice cakes.

### OR

### Carrot and Celery Sticks

Carrot and Celery Sticks
Serve with 50g of hummus.

### OR

### Avocado or Ricotta Crispbread

Spread a little avocado onto 1 or 2 vegan crispbread slices.
Top with sliced tomato, olives and a few pine nuts
Have with one cup of fat burning matcha green tea or of liver cleansing dandelion tea.

Dandelion tea is a great weight loss hack, it helps to reduce fluid retention whilst also acting as a liver cleanser.
The bitter qualities help to reduce cravings and will assist with skin conditions as it aids liver function.

# Dinner

### Grilled Tofu / Tempeh or Vegan Meat Burger

Grill or lightly fry in olive oil a small piece, 150g or less, and have together with one to two cups of steamed green vegetables or with a small portion of sweet potato fries. The vegetables can be dressed with a little olive oil and garlic, sea salt or black pepper.

### OR

### Squash and Lentil Stew

Add a cup of pre-cooked lentils in sachet or tin to quarter of a cup of diced butternut squash to water.
Simmer slowly and add turmeric, chilli, garlic and ginger.
Serve on a bed of brown rice in a small bowl.

### OR

### Green Vegetable and Cauliflower Stir Fry

Stir fry a cupful of green vegetables and cauliflower with a 100/150g of tempeh, tofu or vegan meat substitute pieces.
Season with spices of choice - tamari works well here as does vegetable seasoning.
Half a cup of brown rice can be added to increase healthy wholegrain intake.

# After Dinner

### Dates or Prunes with Rice or Almond Milk

2 or 3 dates or prunes; served warm with a splash of unsweetened rice or almond milk.

# Before Bed

### Herbal Tea

1 cup of herbal tea; choose calming varieties like chamomile, lemon balm or valerian.

# Exercises for **Weeks 1&3**

## Warm Up
### 1 Minute Cardio – Jog

Start by 'walking on the spot' then take it into a jog.
After 30 seconds start to increase intensity and go
as fast as you can, only taking your feet off the floor
a couple of cms (or inches) and moving your arms
fast as well until you hit the minute mark.

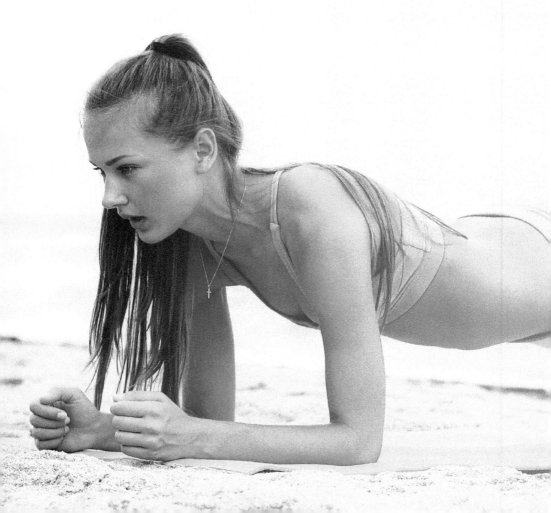

# HIIT Circuit Weeks 1&3

Do each exercise in the circuit for 20 seconds intensely and then slowly for 40 seconds except for the Plank – this should be held for 20 seconds and then relaxed for 40 seconds at the beginner level. Each individual exercise within the circuit should be done for 1 minute with a one minute rest in between circuits. Rest for one minute after each circuit.

**Beginner** – complete once or twice
**Intermediate** – complete two or three times
**Advanced** – complete three or four times

These can be done two to three times per week and can be combined with two days of LISS workouts. The LISS workout can be a twenty minute brisk walk.

## Speed Squats

Stand with feet hip width apart and lower the hips down in a squat as if you're sitting on a low chair, sticking out your butt behind you. Move quickly back to a standing position and repeat.

As you squat down keep arms straight but raise them to parallel with the floor as you squat down.

Keep the timing steady.

## Plank

Start by getting into a push up position.

**Beginners** – on knees / elbows

**Intermediate** – on toes / hands

**Advanced** – move from elbows to hands and alternate from one to the other keeping the core activated at all times.

Bend your elbows and rest your weight onto your forearms or hands.

Engage your core by pulling your belly button in towards your spine.

To increase the intensity of the intermediate move, lift 1 leg by 5cms from the floor and then lower and change.

Alternate legs every 5 seconds.

### Static Running

Assume Running Position, with one leg forward, one back – as if about to start a race.

Bend your arms and move them back and forth quickly as if you are running very fast.

Increase the speed of the movement to increase the intensity and to raise the heart rate.

### Abs – Leg Raise & Touch Toes

Lie on your back with your shoulders on the floor and your legs straight up in the air.

Breathe in.

As you exhale reach your hands towards toes, lifting shoulders away from the ground.

Touch your toes if possible and pulse.

## Stretch & Relax

Seated forward bend.

Sit down with your legs flat and straight out in front of you.

Breathe in, raise hands to the ceiling and slowly lean forward keeping your back straight initially.

Hold this position reaching as far towards your toes as you can. Either hold hands around your feet, or use a small towel around your feet to draw yourself further into the stretch.

Aim to hold this position for 1 minute, or longer.

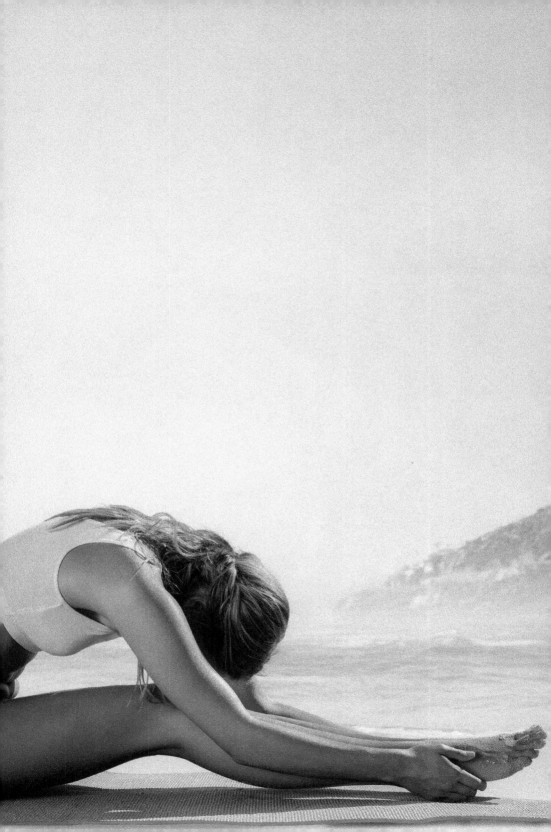

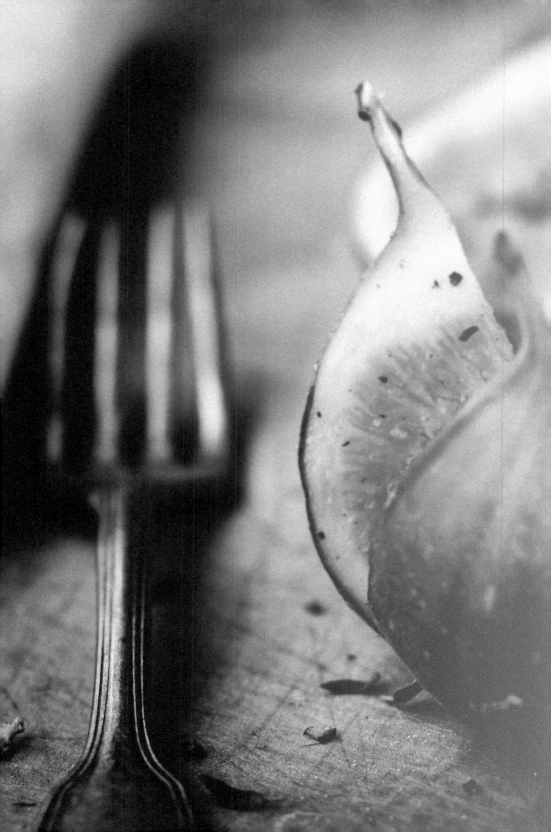

# Weeks
# 2&4

# Balance

## Before Breakfast
### Grapefruit Blast

Half a glass of warm filtered water with the juice of half a grapefruit to kick start the liver and gallbladder and digestive function.

This early morning combination helps with fat metabolism also. This liver tonic will also help regulate blood sugar levels and diminish cravings.

Add cinnamon if desired to further help reduce cravings.

# Breakfast

For weeks 2 and 4 make sure that there is a twelve to fourteen hour window between dinner or dessert and breakfast.

### Green Mango Smoothie

• 1 cup frozen mango • ½ apple • 1 cup organic spinach • 4-5 fresh mint leaves • 1 inch fresh peeled ginger and 2 teaspoons fresh lemon juice.

Blend in 200 mls of water.

### OR

### Strawberry Maca Smoothie Bowl

Blend • 1 cup frozen strawberries • ½ cup coconut yogurt • ¼ cup almond milk and 1 tsp maca powder

Transfer to a small bowl and top with buckwheat granola, sliced strawberries, blueberries, sliced almonds and a few sunflower seeds.

Go easy on the toppings just a little of each ingredient.

### OR

### Raspberry Smoothie

Blend • two cups of raspberries • one cup of spinach • one teaspoon cinnamon and two teaspoons chia or linseeds in 200 mls of hemp • rice • oat • or almond milk.

You can boost your shake by adding 1 scoop of plant based protein.

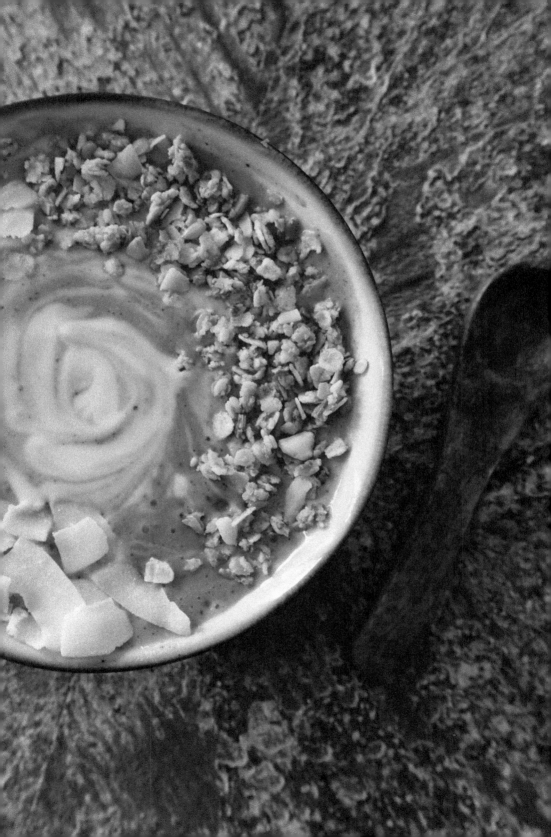

# Snack

### Fruit and Nuts Yogurt Treat

1 Banana or apple; with a few almonds and a few teaspoons of coconut yogurt if desired.

Eating every few hours helps to control portion size and helps to regulate blood sugar levels thereby reducing cravings and helping with mood and cognitive performance.

**OR**

### Cashew Nut Fruit Bowl

1 Small bowl portion of fruit salad; with a few cashew nuts.

Berries, apples, pears and melons are recommended.

**OR**

### Brown Rice Cakes

2 Rice cakes with avocado or nut butter – almond or cashew preferably.

This snack is rich in antioxidants and healthy omegas.

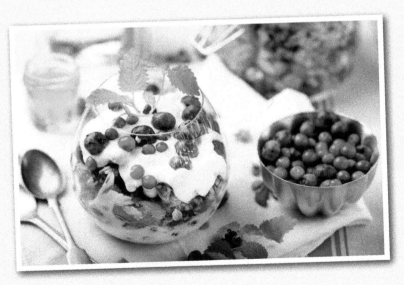

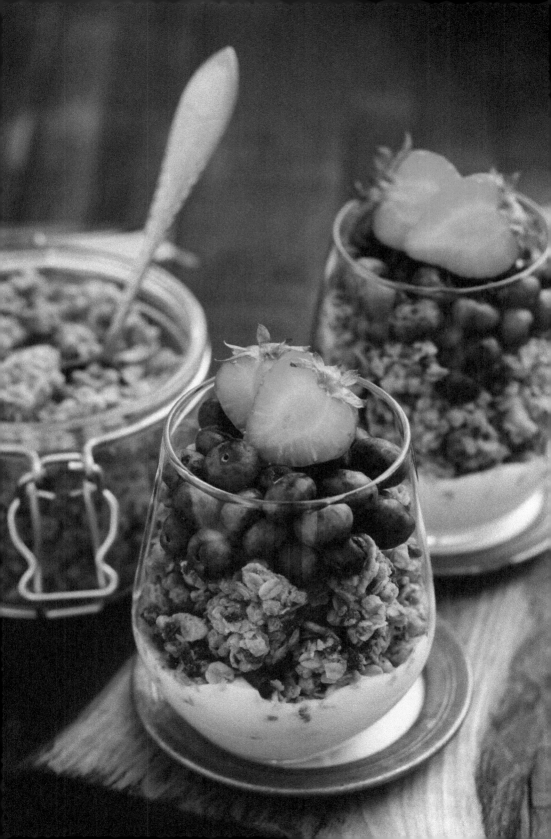

# Before Lunch & Dinner

### Spirulina Super Green Boost

3 to 6 Spirulina or Super Green tablets can be taken as they help with feelings of fullness and with controlling portion size. They also help to alkalise and detox the system.

# Lunch

### Chilli Chickpeas/ Mixed Beans with Vegan Burger

Grill or lightly fry in olive oil one vegan burger and serve with a cup of chilli chick peas or mixed beans – add a teaspoon of olive oil, balsamic vinegar and a little chilli or cayenne to the chick peas.

This protein based meal is high in antioxidants to boost immunity and is rich in healthy omegas to help with mood, cognition and skin conditions.

## OR

### Green Pesto with Basil Wholewheat Penne

For the pesto blend 2 cups fresh basil leaves, ½ cup extra virgin olive oil, 1/3 cup of pine nuts together with 2 garlic cloves, ¼ teaspoon of sea or rock salt, 1/8 teaspoon freshly ground black pepper and 2 tablespoons of water.

Boil a cupful of wholewheat or lentil pasta until al dente - around 12 minutes.

Serve with a side salad of a bowl of mixed green leaves topped with a little balsamic vinegar.

## OR

### Vegan Stir Fry

Lightly fry in olive oil two cups of mixed vegetables, such as courgette, mushrooms, carrots, green beans and spinach with one teaspoon of grated fresh ginger.

Add in a handful of cashew nuts when the vegetables are almost ready.

Add mood boosting turmeric and sesame seeds. Serve with rice noodles or brown rice.

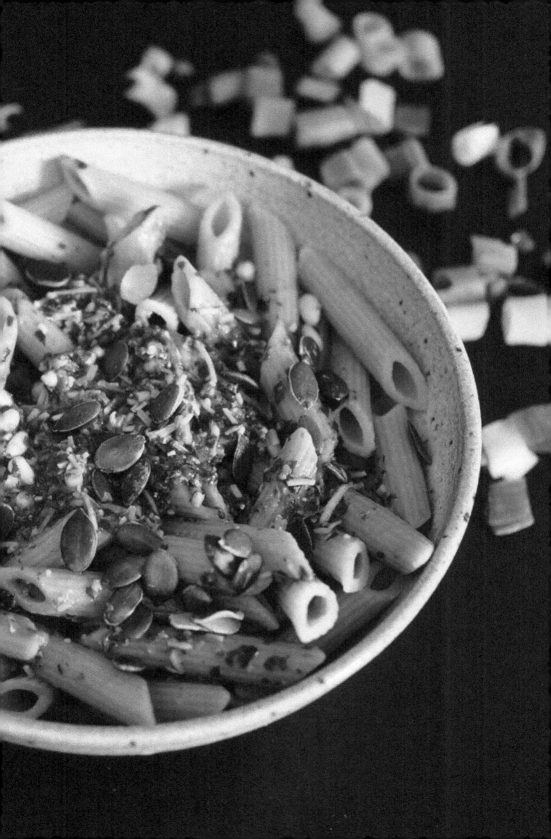

# Mid Afternoon

### Date or Prune Nut Mix

4 or 5 Dried dates or prunes; with 2 or 3 teaspoons of mixed nuts or seeds.

### OR

### Seeds, Nuts and Apple

2 or 3 Teaspoons of mixed nuts and seeds with half an apple.

### OR

### Carrot and Apple Juice

One fresh carrot, ginger and apple juice.

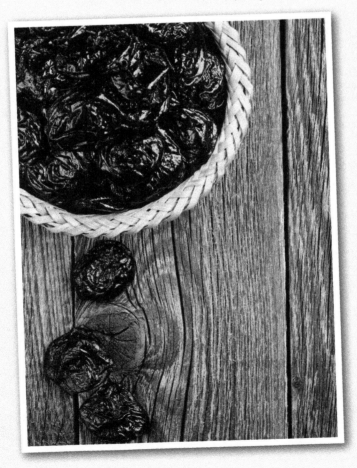

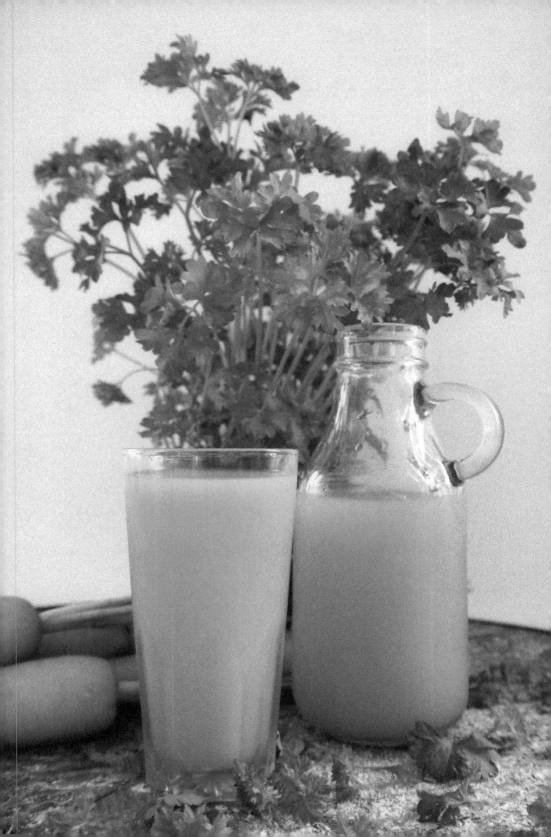

# Dinner

### Miso Mushroom Soup

Heat and lightly simmer for 10 to 15 minutes:
• 500 mls miso stock • 50g chestnut mushrooms • 4 sliced spring onions, 50g broccoli florets • 4 pieces of baby corn • a few thin slices of fresh red chilli and 2 tbsp chopped fresh coriander.

Season to taste with soy sauce or use a little sea or salt and black pepper.

### OR

### Cauliflower Soup

Blend • 1 garlic clove • 1 chopped onion • 4 or 5 cauliflower florets • 6 or 7 cashews • a teaspoon of turmeric • a teaspoon of chilli and a pinch of sea salt and black pepper.

Pour into saucepan and add 350 mls of filtered water and ½ veggie stock cube. Cook for 1 minute, then simmer gently for fifteen minutes.

Top with some grated vegan cheese.

### OR

### Broccoli, Green Beans and Spinach Stir Fry

Stir fry a cup of broccoli and one of green beans in olive oil. Season with spices of choice and serve with half a cup of brown rice.

Lightly stir fry one cup of broccoli and one of green beans in coconut oil. Season with tamari and spices of choice.

Top with a handful or two of almonds and serve with half a cup of brown rice.

# After Dinner

### Cacao Milk

Warm a cup of unsweetened rice or almond milk slowly.

Add a teaspoon of 100% raw cacao and a hint of chilli powder to help burn fat if desired.

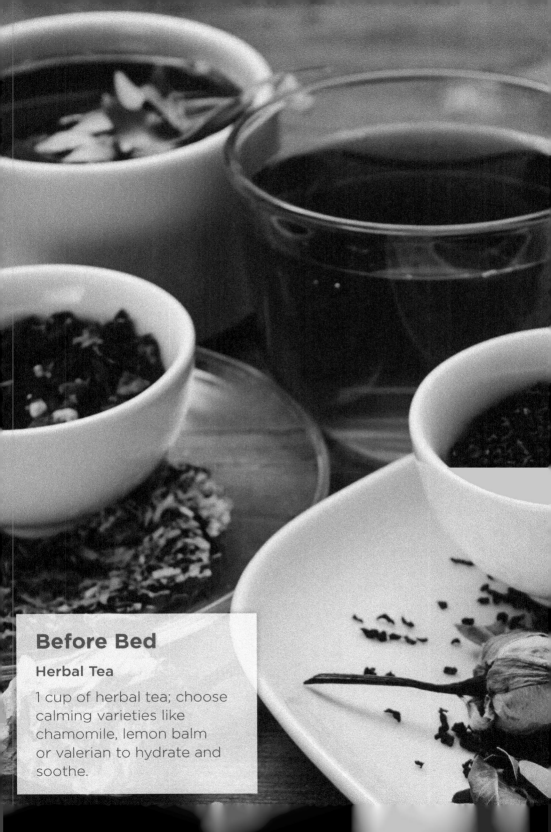

## Before Bed

### Herbal Tea

1 cup of herbal tea; choose calming varieties like chamomile, lemon balm or valerian to hydrate and soothe.

# Exercises for **Weeks 2 & 4**

## Warm Up
### 1 Minute Cardio – Knee Raise

Hold your hands out in front of you and lift your knees toward your hands one at a time, then take it into a jog and raise the hands until they are parallel to the floor, touching your knees to your hands if possible.
To increase intensity increase the speed and the height of the knees.
To engage the oblique muscles (side core) more go back to a walking speed.
Take your knee toward the opposite elbow with your hands placed behind your head and alternate.

## HIIT Circuit Weeks 2&4

Do each exercise in the circuit for 20 seconds intensely and then slowly for 40 seconds.

Each individual exercise within the circuit should be done for 1 minute.

Rest for one minute after each circuit.

Do this HIIT circuit two to three times per week.

For your LISS workout walk, swim or cycle at medium pace for twenty five minutes twice week.

**Beginner** – complete once or twice
**Intermediate** – complete two or three times
**Advanced** – complete three or four times

### Superman
Come down onto all fours.
Activate core by drawing in the belly button towards the spine.

Stretch forward your right arm, and outstretch your left leg, keeping them parallel to the floor, hold for 5 seconds then repeat with your opposite arm and leg till you reach your chosen time level.

## Mountain Climbers

Assume a high plank position (on hands and toes). Make sure the shoulders are positioned over the wrists.

From here draw one knee at a time towards the nose and return to the start position.

Perform this movement quickly as if you were 'running'. Keep the hips low.

To activate the oblique muscles (side core) take the knee toward the opposite elbow as you move it forward.

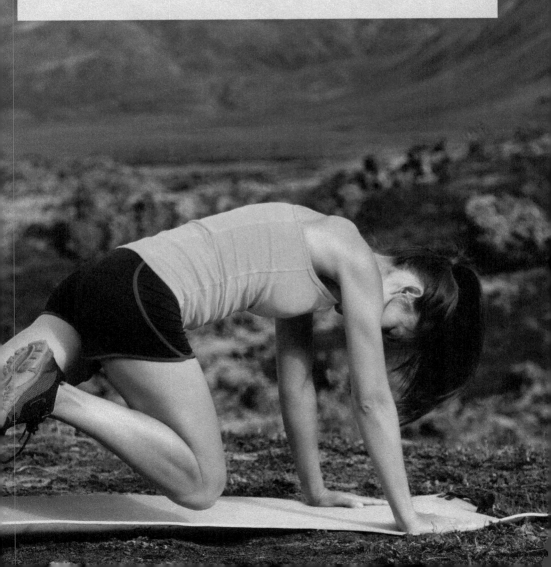

## Squat with Shoulder Press

Just hands only or light weights.

Start in a standing position and go down to a low squat with your hands at shoulder level and with your arms outstretched to the side keeping your elbows bent.

As you stand, move the hands (with weights) straight up overhead.

Squat and repeat.

## Abs – Elbow to Knee (Obliques)

Slow motion.

Lying down, raise your lower legs to a tabletop position (lower legs parallel to floor), with your hands held behind supporting your head.

Rotate your elbow to the opposite knee as you stretch out the other leg and repeat.

Keep your shoulders off the floor at all times to engage the abdominals.

# Stretch & Relax
### Child's Pose

Sit on your heels and place your knees either together or apart (i.e. towards the edge of your yoga mat).

Sitting back onto your heels walk your hands forwards.

Keep your bottom on your heels and stretch out placing the forearms on the mat ahead of you.

Lower your head to the mat.
This primarily stretches your lower back, hips and knees.

Hold for at least 1 minute.

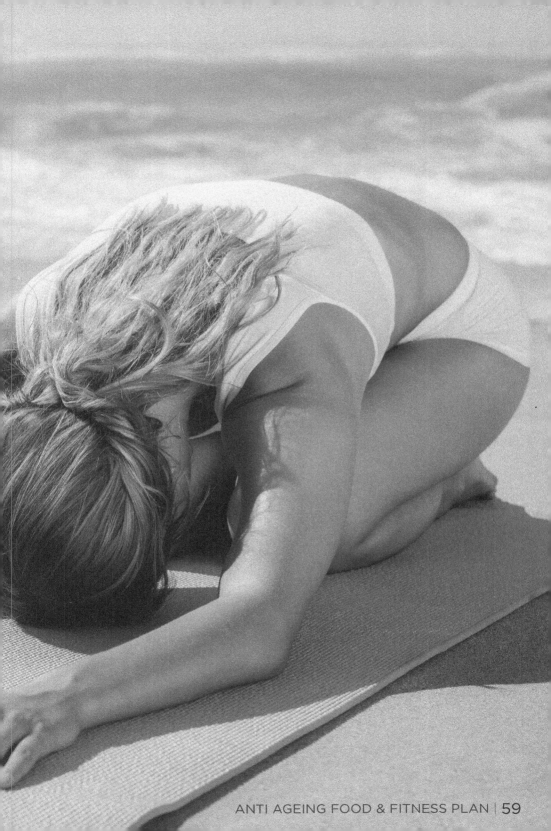

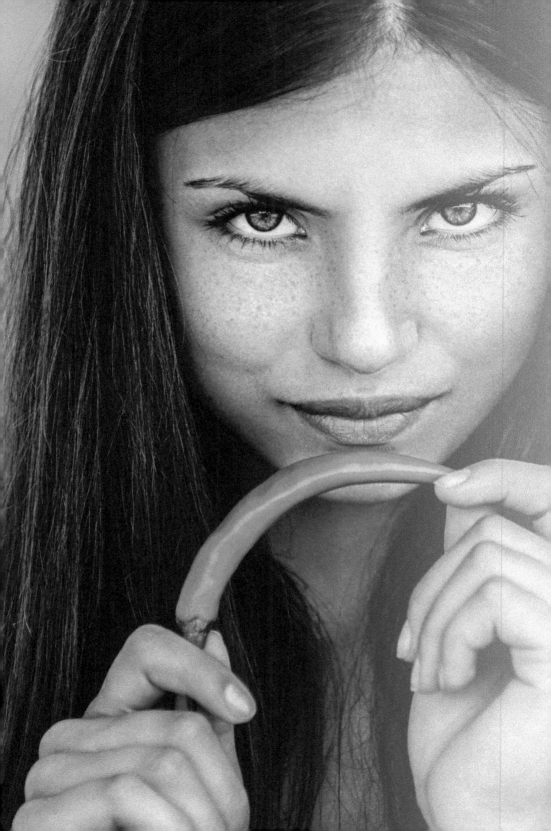

# Intro Weeks 5 to 8

You should have noticed some changes already in weight reduction and fitness levels.
The condition of your skin should have also improved along with positive changes in body shape.

During weeks 5 to 8 the plan continues to use thermogenic spices such as cayenne, chilli, pepper and turmeric to assist with the metabolism of fat from the body.

The blood sugar regulating super spice, cinnamon, is also recommended throughout this four week period to help reduce cravings and to assist with weight management.

Weeks 5 to 8 see you continue to gently cleanse the system with high fibre main meal, snack and dessert options.

One important thing to consider at this point are your stress levels. Make sure that you are getting adequate rest.

Stress can be very damaging to the body and can exacerbate any underlying conditions - it also is linked to increased inflammation and negatively impacts immune function.
Chronic stress is also ageing to the body and may even shorten telomeres.
If you are feeling overly anxious or mentally exhausted you might like to try taking a magnesium supplement or one that contains B complex vitamins.
Herbs like St John's Wort, Lemon Balm, Ashwagandha, Siberian Ginseng, Holy Basil and Vervain also provide nervous system support.
Additionally, Reishi and Chaga mushrooms may offer support whilst helping to increase energy levels.

During weeks 5 to 8 if you need more of an energy boost you can have an extra fresh fruit and vegetable juice.

I like one that has beetroot, berries, coconut water and ginger as this helps with nitric oxide production which in turn can help exercise performance.
You should be able to increase your effort in the fitness sections this month too.
Remember to stay hydrated throughout the program.

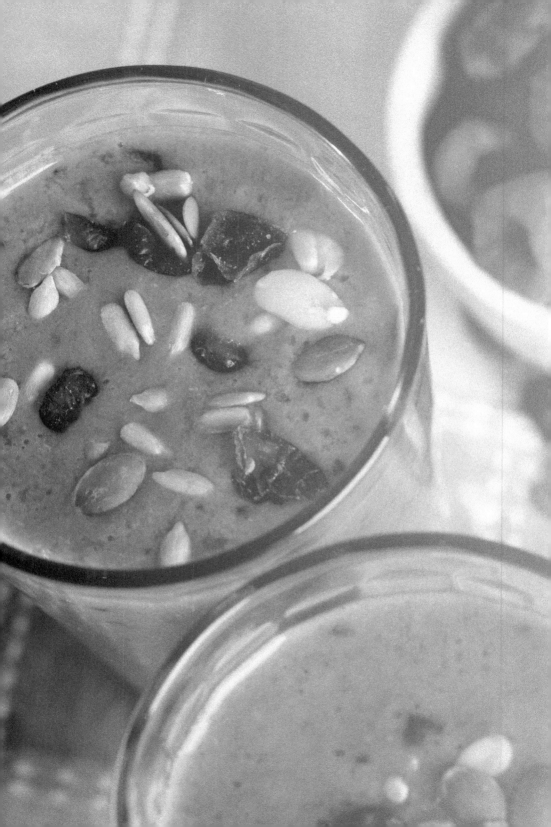

# Weeks
# 5 & 7

# Recharge

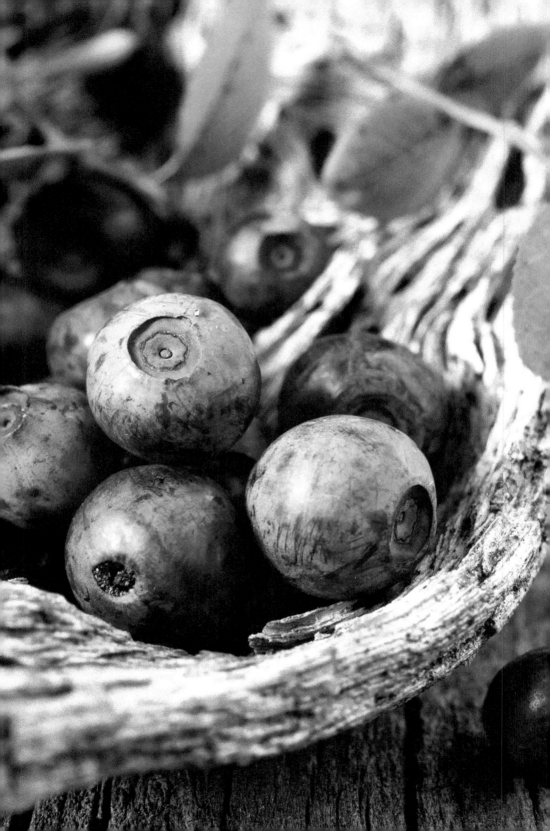

## Before Breakfast

### Lemon Blast

Half a glass of warm filtered water with the juice of half a lemon.

This will kickstart the liver and gallbladder and assist with digestive function.

Add a teaspoon of cinnamon to help reduce cravings and steady mood.

# Breakfast

### Blueberry Protein Smoothie

Blend or blast 1 scoop of Plant Based Protein Powder with 250 mls of unsweetened rice or almond milk and a cup of blueberries.

Add 7 or 8 almonds to increase satiety if desired.

This nutritional blast is now used as a meal replacement. It is high in protein and amino acids to help keep you fuller for longer and will assist in energy production.

A handful of spinach can also be used to increase magnesium levels.

### OR

### Overnight Buckwheat Porridge

• ¼ cup buckwheat groats • 1 tbsp chia seeds • 1 cup unsweetened rice milk • ½ cup water and a pinch of cinnamon.

Mix buckwheat groats, chia seeds, rice milk, water and cinnamon in a bowl or glass container. Cover and let it sit overnight in the fridge.

In the morning place it in a pot, and cook, stirring occasionally, for 15 minutes or until it reaches your desired thickness.

Add a few slices of apple and a little nut butter or some nuts of your choice.

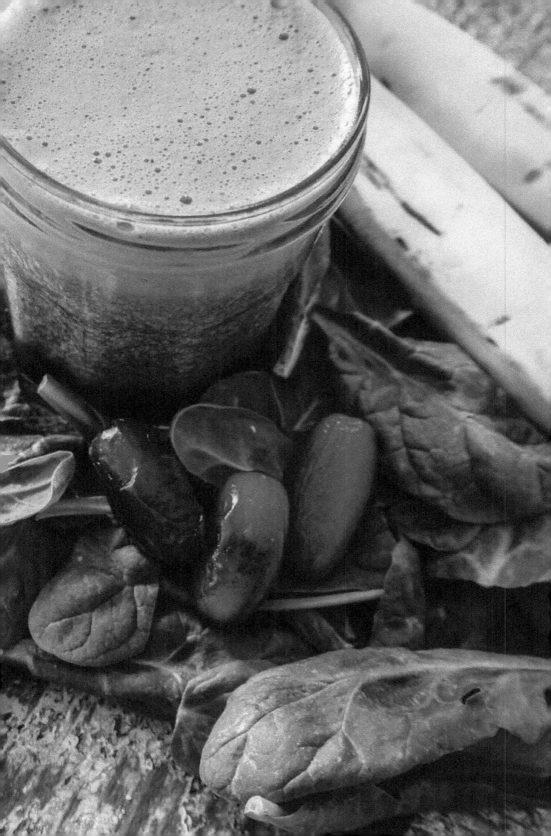

# Mid Morning

## Seasonal Small Nutty Fruit Bowl

Top a small bowl of seasonal fruit with 5 or 6 almonds or cashews. Can be served with a dollop of unsweetened organic soya yogurt.

The fruit and nuts are nutrient dense and help with both cognitive and immune function – the nuts provide protein to help with fullness.

## OR

## Apple and Pecans

1 Apple with 6 to 8 pecans.

## OR

## Omega Density Juice

Blend or blast 7 cashews or almonds with 1 teaspoon of chia seeds, linseeds and sesame seeds.

Add 1 cup of leafy greens and half an avocado and half a banana.

Add a glass of water or coconut water.

This immune booster is high in phytonutrients and is packed full of enzymes for anti ageing cellular health.

The seeds are rich in healthy omegas to promote hair, skin and nail health.
These omegas also assist with cognitive function and weight management.

## AND

## Coffee, Tea or Dandelion Tea

1 Cup of coffee or tea if desired.

This is a great time of day to maximise the fat burning qualities of caffeine.

Do not sweeten with sugar or artificial sweeteners.

The dandelion tea option is good to help reduce bloating and fluid retention.

It also stimulates liver function.

Matcha green tea is another option here.

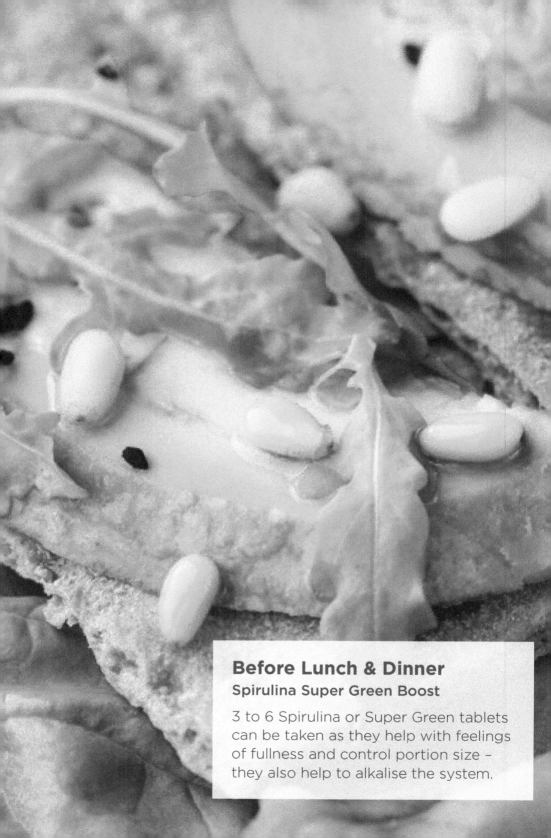

### Before Lunch & Dinner
Spirulina Super Green Boost

3 to 6 Spirulina or Super Green tablets can be taken as they help with feelings of fullness and control portion size – they also help to alkalise the system.

# Lunch

## Warm Beetroot and Spinach Salad with Vegan Feta

• 2 cups of fresh spinach • 1 trimmed beetroot • 1 tbsp minced shallot • ½ tbsp minced fresh parsley • 1 tbsp extra-virgin olive oil, ½ tbsp balsamic vinegar • salt and pepper to taste and 1 tbsp of crumbled vegan feta cheese.

Wash and trim the beetroot, but do not peel.

Place the beetroot in a large saucepan and cover with 2cm of water.

Bring to the boil over high heat, then reduce the heat to medium-low, cover and simmer until just tender, about 30 mins.

Peel the beetroot and cut into 6mm slices.

While the beetroot is cooking whisk together the shallot, parsley, olive oil, balsamic vinegar and red wine vinegar in a bowl until blended; season to taste with salt and pepper, and set aside.

To assemble the dish, place spinach and the warm, sliced beetroots onto a serving dish, pour vinaigrette over the beetroot and sprinkle with vegan feta cheese.

## OR

## Tofu with Salad Greens

Lightly fry a small bowl of tofu in coconut oil.

Serve with a cup sized portion of asparagus, salad greens and broccoli together with 3 or 4 small tomatoes.

Add olive oil, balsamic vinegar and fresh cracked black pepper.

## OR

## Avocado and Black Pepper Vegan Crispbread

Top 2 or 3 crispbreads with half an avocado, black pepper, a few pine nuts and a few olives.

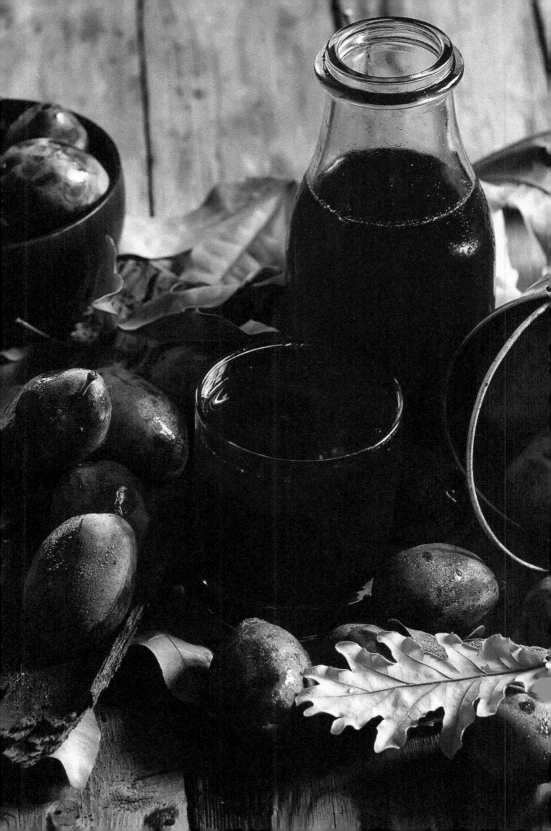

# Mid Afternoon

### Prune Snack with Nuts

3 or 4 Prunes or a glass of unsweetened organic prune juice with one banana.

If you're constipated it's harder to lose weight so regularity is important.

This snack is a great help with energy – both physical and mental.

Have with 2 teaspoons of mixed nuts and seeds for protein to help keep you satisfied till dinner.

## OR

### Pecan / Walnut Fruit Bowl

Small mixed fruit bowl with 6 or 7 pecans or walnuts – any combination of fruits although berries are best.

## OR

### Peppermint or Spearmint Tea

One cup of peppermint or spearmint tea – to calm and stimulate digestion.

Have with a handful of pumpkin or sunflower seeds to provide essential fatty acids.

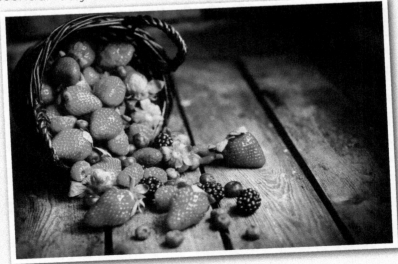

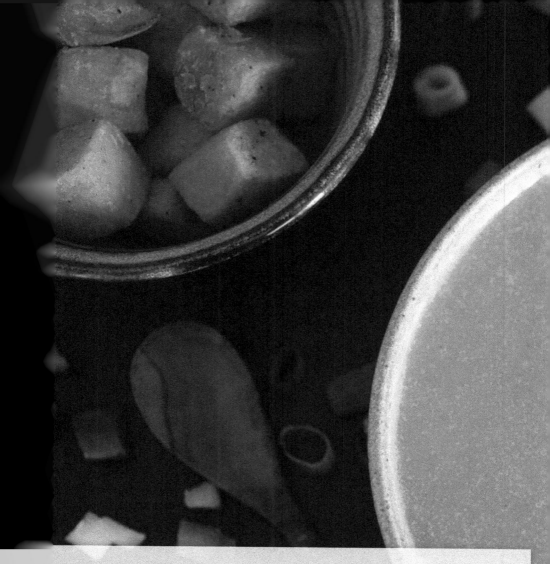

# Dinner

**Carrot and Coconut Soup**

• 3 peeled and chopped carrots • ½ medium chopped onion
• 2 cups vegetable stock • ½ can unsweetened coconut milk
• sea salt • freshly ground black pepper and 2 tablespoons
chilli sauce.

Blend all of the ingredients and add to a saucepan drizzled in
about a tablespoon of cold pressed olive oil.

Cook for approx 20 minutes and top with a teaspoon of
turmeric and a few slivers of almonds or some pine nuts.

**OR**

### Cashew and Pine Nut Vegetable Stir Fry

Stir fry 2 cups of a vegetable medley of your choice in coconut oil.

When ready add 5 or 6 cashews, a handful of pine nuts and a tablespoon of nutritional yeast.

Make sure you add spices to taste as they stimulate the digestive process and speed up metabolism – use soy sauce, ginger, chilli and garlic.

Can be served with a small cup of brown rice.

**OR**

### Sweet Potato, Pea and Spinach Soup

• ½ onion • chopped, 1 tbsp olive oil • 2 cloves garlic • ¼ small sweet potato - peeled and chopped • 350ml vegan vegetable stock • handful of frozen peas • handful of spinach and a dollop of soya cream.

Gently fry the onion in the oil, add the garlic and sweet potato, continue to cook for another 5 minutes.

Add the stock to the pan and simmer for 15 minutes or until the sweet potato is cooked. Add the peas and spinach to the pan and simmer for 10 minutes.

Let the soup cool for a few minutes then blend until smooth.

Add the soya cream and serve.

**AND**

### Dandelion Tea / Coffee

• 1 Cup of herbal tea • such as unsweetened dandelion • fennel • fenugreek or liquorice.

Dandelion's bitter qualities aid liver function making it good for weight loss, fluid retention, bloating and skin conditions.

Fennel and fenugreek are both digestive tonics whilst liquorice is an adrenal tonic and energy booster.

Fat burning matcha green tea is another option here.

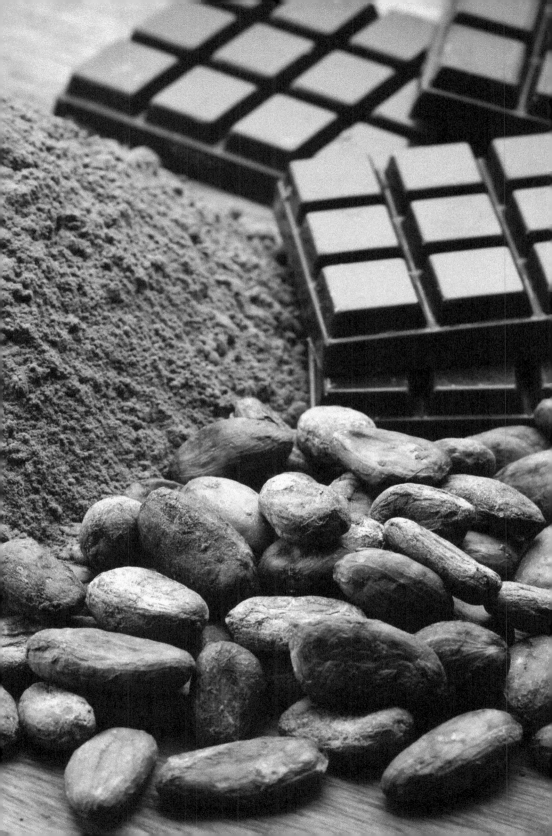

# After Dinner

### Cacao treat

1 Teaspoon of cacao with 250 mls of unsweetened rice or almond milk.

This can be served hot or cold.

Have with a handful of nuts and dried fruits if desired as they will help to stabilise mood and satisfy a sweet tooth.

Half a teaspoon of chilli powder can be added to help with lymphatic function and fat burning.

### OR

Vegan Chocolate Squares and Almonds
2 Squares of vegan chocolate and 5 or 6 almonds.

# Before Bed

### Calming Herbal Tea

1 Cup of herbal tea – choose a calming variety like chamomile, lemon balm or valerian.

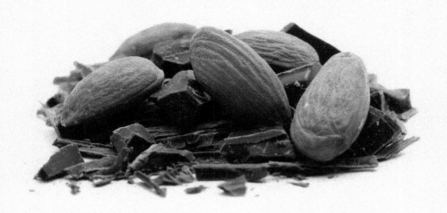

# Exercises for **Weeks 5&7**

## Warm Up
### 1 Minute Cardio – Glute Reverse Kicks

Start in a jog, then place your hands behind your bottom, palms facing out and begin to kick your heels into your hands – for approx 30 seconds.

Change direction and place your arms out in front of you and start to kick your feet toward the opposite hand – again for 30 seconds and try to touch your toes.

## HIIT Circuit Weeks 5&7

Do each exercise in the circuit for 30 seconds intensely and then slowly for 30 seconds except for the Side Plank – this should be held for 30 seconds and then relaxed for 30 seconds.

Each individual exercise within the circuit should be done for 1 minute. Rest for one minute after each exercise too.

**Beginner** – complete once or twice

**Intermediate** – complete two or three times

**Advanced** – complete three or four times

Complete this circuit three or four times per week

Combine this with 30 minutes of LISS exercise - this can be steady walking, cycling or swimming.

## Lunge with Bicep Curl

Start standing straight.

Take one big step forward lowering your back knee to the ground taking your front knee over the ankle as you perform a bicep curl.

Push back to standing and alternate legs. Don't take your knee past your ankle.

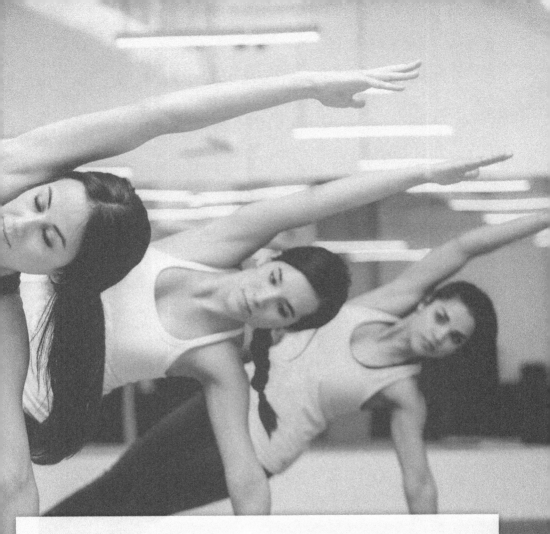

## Side Plank

Lie on your side then place your hand on the floor, directly under your shoulder, and raise your body to a Side Plank (straight) position.

If you have issues with your wrists, this can be done on your elbow.

Hold this static pose for half of your allotted time frame, then turn and do the opposite side.

To increase the intensity do small pulsing movements raising the hips toward the ceiling – only by about 5 cms or 2½ inches.

## Burpee / Jump back then stand

Start in standing position.

Take your hands flat to the floor assuming a crouch position.

Jump the legs back to a high plank pose then return to standing and repeat.

To increase intensity do an actual Burpee, where you jump in the air (rather then just going to a standing position) add in a push up after the jump back.

## Abs – Heel Tap

Lay down on your back with your knees in a bent position and your heels near your bottom.

Lift your shoulders slightly away from the floor, engage abs and reach one hand down by your side to tap your heel.

Repeat and alternate. Aim to keep shoulders off the floor, and don't hold your breath!

# Stretch & Relax

### Seated tree pose

Sit down with one leg stretched straight out in front of you with your foot flexed and place your other foot at your inner thigh.

Sit up tall with a long, straight spine and neutral neck, breathe in and raise the hands in the air.

Lean forward over the extended leg with your hands towards your foot.

Either hold onto the foot and draw yourself further forward or again use a small towel to achieve this.

Reverse and repeat on the other side.

Hold for at least 1 minute and move with the breath by sinking deeper into the stretch with each exhalation.

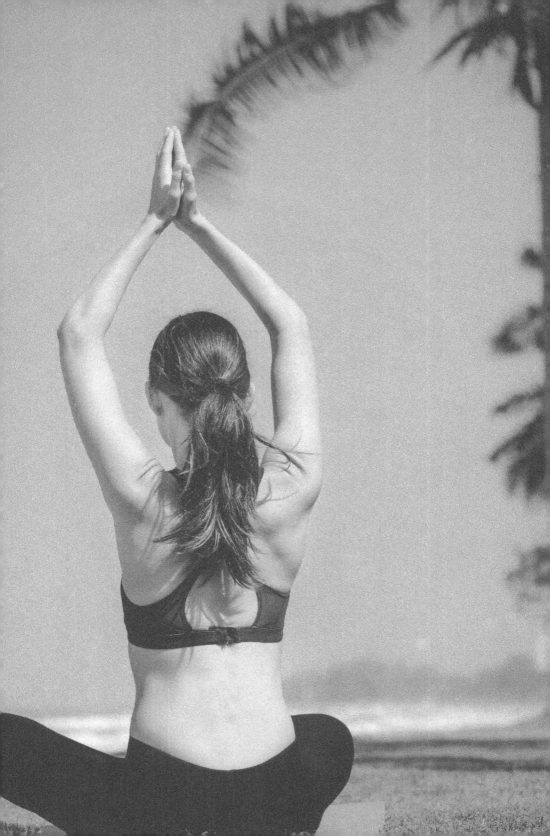

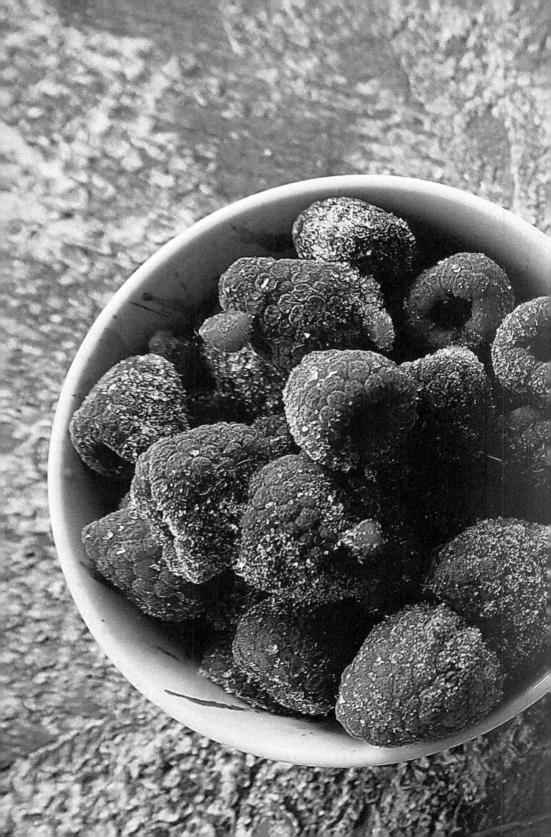

# Weeks
# 6&8

# Recharge

For weeks 6 and 8 do not eat breakfast early.

Try to leave a twelve to fourteen hour window between dinner or dessert and breakfast.

# Breakfast

### Blueberry, Rhubarb and Apple Porridge

Add 3 tablespoons of antioxidant rich blueberries, stewed rhubarb or stewed apples to a small bowl of porridge. The oats help keep blood sugar levels stable and assist with cravings whilst the fruit helps to keep your immune system strong.

This breakfast is both calming and stimulating to the digestive tract.

### OR

### Raspberry Smoothie

Blend 250 mls of unsweetened rice or almond milk with a cup of fresh or frozen raspberries.

Add 1 scoop of Plant Based Protein.
Then add 5 or 6 almonds to promote satiety.

### OR

### Small Mixed Berry Bowl

Have 1 cup of fresh or frozen berries with a dollop of coconut yogurt.

Top with 5 or 6 almonds.

The berries are phytonutrient dense superfood option that help keep your immune system strong whilst the nuts povide some protein to help keep you full and focused.

### AND

### Tea, Coffee or Herbal Tea

1 cup of coffee, tea or herbal tea of choice to help with fullness and hydration.

The caffeine in the coffee has fat burning qualities but choose a calming herbal tea if anxiety is an issue.

You might like to have Matcha Green Tea or Yerba Mate to assist with weight loss goals.

Do not add sugar or artificial sweeteners.

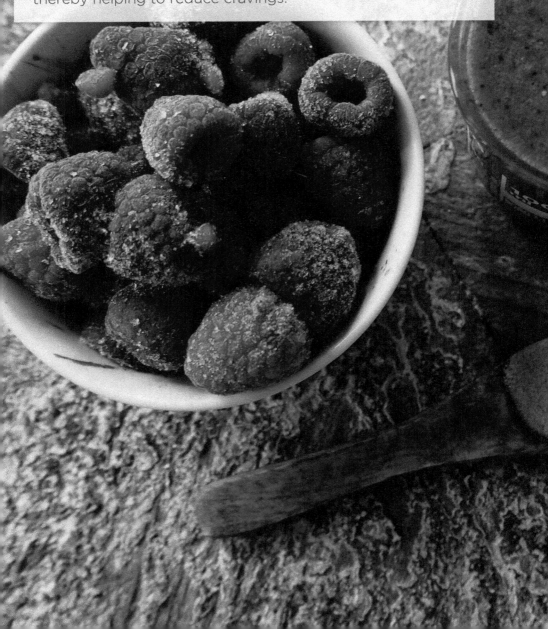

## Before Breakfast
### Grapefruit Blast

One glass or cup of warm filtered water with the juice of half a grapefruit and a little cinnamon to kick start digestion and fat metabolism.

This morning combination also regulates blood sugar levels thereby helping to reduce cravings.

# Snack

### Dates, Nut and Seed Mix

Have 3 or 4 dates to help with regularity – if you're not regular it's harder to lose weight.

Also have 3 teaspoons of mixed nuts and seeds as the protein content will keep you satisfied.

### OR

### Almonds and Apple

1 Apple with 8 – 10 almonds is the prefect snack to promote fullness.

The pectin in the apple combines perfectly with the protein in the nuts to ensure satiety.

### OR

### Herbal Tea

1 Cup of herbal tea
Spearmint or Peppermint both aid digestive function.

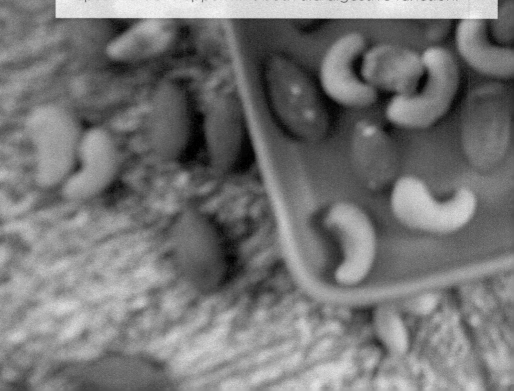

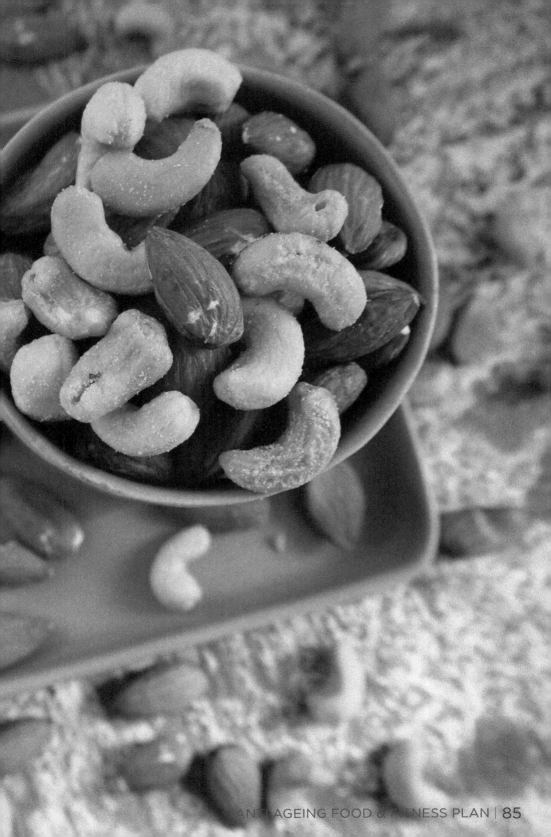

## Before Lunch & Dinner

### Before Lunch & Dinner

Spirulina Super Green Boost

3 to 6 Spirulina or Super Green tablets can be taken as they help with feelings of fullness and to control portion size.

If you prefer powders make a supergreen shot.

These greens help to alkalise, detox and cleanse.

# Lunch

### Tahini Roasted Cauliflower

- ¼ small cauliflower • a handful of toasted pumpkin seeds
- 1 tablespoons coriander seeds • ½ tablespoons black peppercorns, 1 tablespoon cumin seeds • ¼ teaspoon nutmeg, 1 tablespoon paprika, 1 teaspoon turmeric • 1 tablespoons tahini • juice from ½ lemon • 2 tablespoons cold pressed olive oil, 1 tablespoon water and ½ teaspoon salt

Preheat oven to 350°F.

Brush oven-proof dish with olive oil.

Bring a large pot of water to boil and cook the cauliflower for 6-8 minutes then drain.

Toast peppercorns, coriander, cumin, and cloves on a hot dry pan, until fragrant.

Remove pan from heat.

Grind spices.

Add the rest of the spices and mix together.

Mix Tahini, oil, spices blend, lemon, water, salt together.

Spread the mixture all over the cauliflower.

Roast cauliflower in the oven for 30 minutes or until it can be pierced easily with a fork. Remove from the oven and garnish with toasted pumpkin seeds.

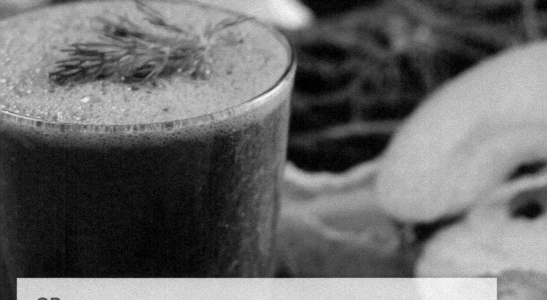

## OR

### Beetroot Salad

• 2 cups of fresh spinach • 2 beetroots trimmed • 1 tbsp minced shallot • 1 tbsp minced fresh parsley • 1 tbsp extra-virgin olive oil • 1 tbsp balsamic vinegar • sea salt and black pepper to taste and 2 tbsp crumbled vegan feta cheese

Wash and trim the beetroots, but do not peel.

Place beetroots in a large saucepan and cover with 3cm of water.

Bring to the boil over high heat, then reduce the heat to medium-low, cover and simmer until just tender for about 30 mins.

Peel beetroots and cut into 6mm slices.

While the beetroot is cooking, whisk together the shallot, parsley, olive oil, balsamic vinegar and red wine vinegar in a bowl.

Season to taste with salt and pepper, and set aside.

To assemble the dish, place the spinach and the warm, sliced beetroots onto a serving dish and pour the vinaigrette over the beetroots.

Sprinkle with vegan feta cheese or vegan cheese.

Can also add pine nuts if desired.

## Mid Afternoon

### Turmeric Latte

Try one to two teaspoons of turmeric in a glass of rice or coconut milk heated in a saucepan with a little agave syrup and some ginger and cinnamon.

### OR

### Carrot or Celery Sticks

Mash half an avocado and serve with 4 or 5 small carrot or celery sticks.

Add cayenne to spice things up.

### AND

### Glass of Kombucha

Have a glass of Kombucha to help with digestive function.

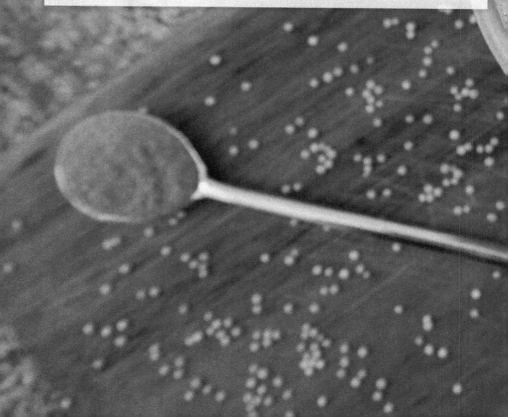

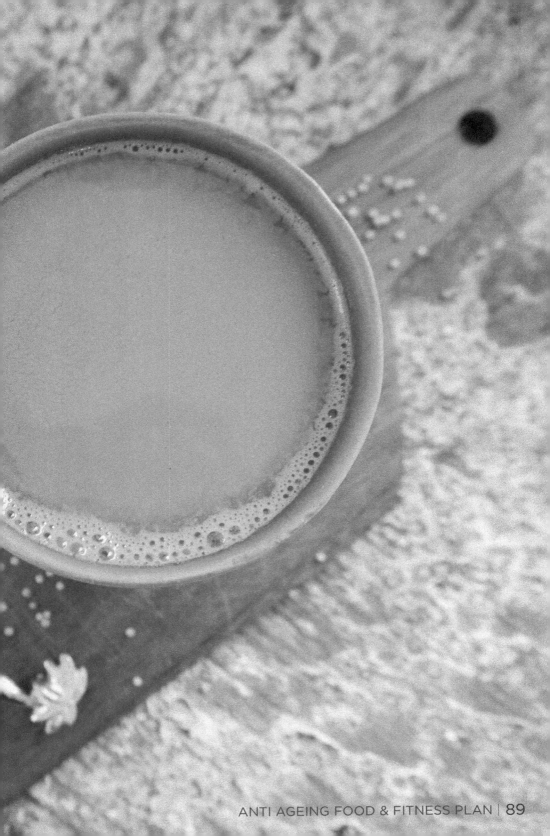

# Dinner

### Vegetable Lentil Soup

Add a cup of pre-cooked lentils or mixed beans and 2 cups of mixed vegetables to 300/400mls of water.

Add ½ cube of vegetable stock and bring to boil. Simmer slowly and add turmeric, chilli and ginger. Have with 1 small slice of wholegrain toast.

Soups are a great choice when on a weight management campaign – they are hydrating, filling and easy on the digestive system.

## OR

### Mediterranean Chilli Roast Vegetables

• 2 cups of any vegetables such as red onion • courgette • peppers and tomatoes.

Bake for 20 minutes in a small lasagne dish with a drizzle of cold pressed olive oil and garlic, herb and chilli seasoning.

You could also add half a cup of lentils or chick peas to increase the protein content of this meal.

## OR

### Smoothie Bowl

• 1 mango • chopped & frozen • ½ frozen banana • ½ cup of coconut yoghurt • ½ cup of nut milk • blueberries • raspberries

Add all ingredients into a high-speed blender. Blend until smooth.

Spoon into a small bowl.

Add berries.

## AND

### Spearmint, Peppermint, Fennel or Dandelion Tea

All of these teas are digestive and liver tonics.

## After Dinner

### Stewed Pears

Stew one pear in a little filtered water and add some sultanas or raisins.

Top with a little cinnamon, chilli or cayenne to regulate blood sugar and boost fat burning.

## Before Bed

### Calming Sleepy Tea

1 Cup of calming herbal tea

Choose either chamomile, lemon balm or valerian to nourish the nervous system.

# Exercises for **Weeks 6&8**

## Warm Up
### 1 Minute Cardio – Jumping Jacks

Begin by simply stepping from side to side raising your hands and arms up above you as you do so.

Then move your arms down again in coordination with your steps.

To increase the intensity start to move the legs out whilst raising the arms at the same time.

Increase speed to intensify further.

## HIIT Circuit Weeks 6&8

Do each exercise in the circuit for 30 seconds intensely and then slowly for 30 seconds.

Each individual exercise within the circuit should be done for 1 minute.

Rest for one minute after each circuit.

**Beginner** – complete once or twice

**Intermediate** – complete two or three times

**Advanced** – complete three or four times

The HIIT circuit should be completed three to four times per week with a further two LISS exercise sessions on other days.

The LISS sessions can be 35 minutes of steady walking, slow jogging, swimming or cycling.

## Reverse Lunge with Toe (High Kick) Touch

Start in a standing position with your hands on your hips.

Take a step back and lower the back knee towards the floor in a lunge position.

Then push off from that back foot to bring that leg forward in front of your body with the knee bent to a 90 degree angle and touch your toes – repeat x5.

Repeat on other side.

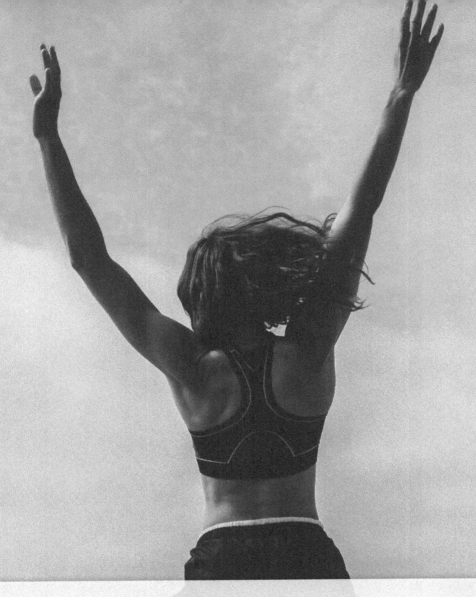

## Bridge with Knee Raise

Lie flat on your back with your knees in a bent knee position with your heels towards your bottom.

Your lower back should be pressed into the floor with a small natural arch at the lower spine to activate the core.

Raise the hips away from the ground to a bridge pose and at the same time lift one knee towards your chest while squeezing the glutes.

Return to the floor and repeat on the other side.

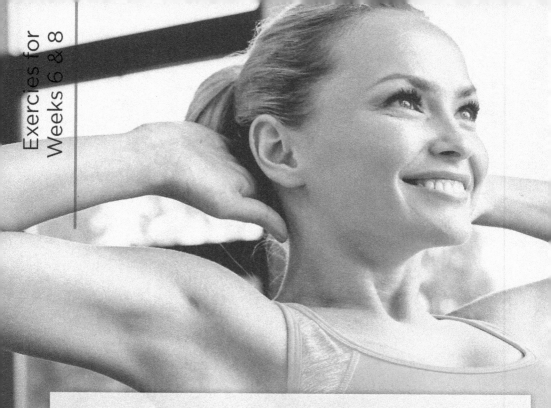

### Roll Down with Push Up

Begin in a standing position with your core engaged.

Start to slide your hands down toward the ground bending your knees until the hands are flat on the floor.

Then walk the hands forward until you are in a high Plank position.

Perform either a full or half push up before walking the hands back and rolling back up to a standing position.

Repeat for allotted time.

### Abs – Crunch

Lay down with your knees bent.
Your feet should hover above ground about 2 cms or 1 inch.

Pull your knees to your chest keeping the calves resting against your hamstrings as you raise your shoulders from the floor to meet your knees.

Make sure you keep your neck neutral and don't bend it forward.

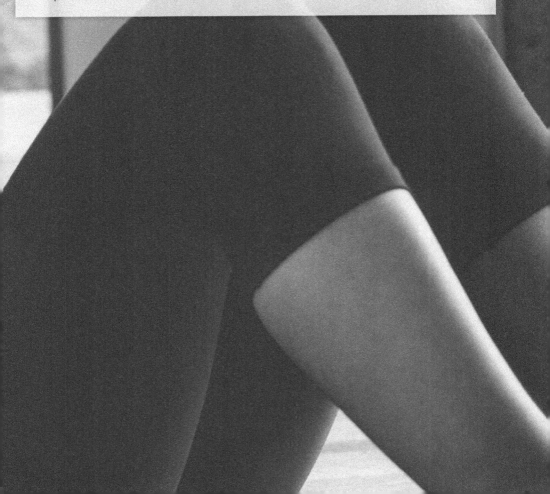

# Stretch & Relax

### Lunge pose into Pyramid pose

Start with the right foot placed between your hands on the floor.

Stretch out your left leg behind you in a lunge or runner's position, stretching out your hip flexor (thigh) and glute.

Hold here for 15 – 20 seconds then straighten the front right leg to form a triangle or pyramid shape with your legs.

Make sure to keep this front leg in a straight position.

Reach you hands down towards the right foot – either have your hands flat on the floor or hold onto your ankle or leg if less flexible.

Repeat on the other side.

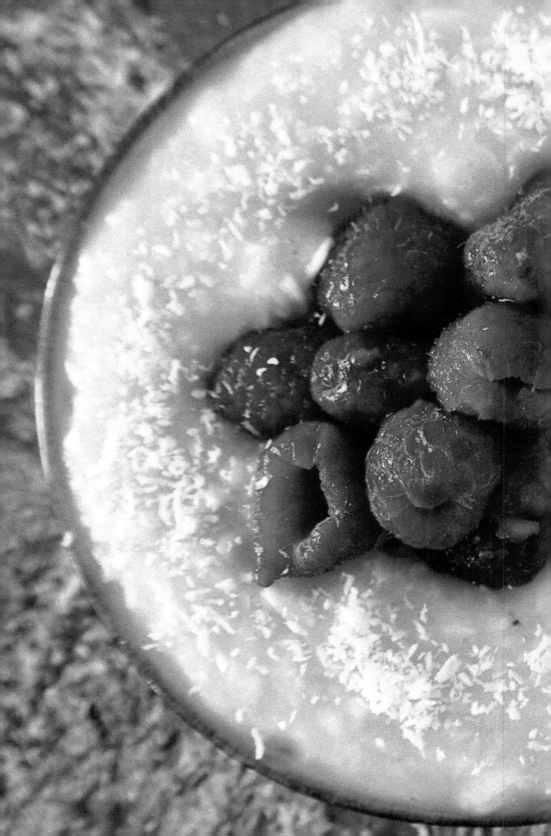

# Intro Weeks 9 to 12

*Congratulations on making it to the final four weeks of your health and fitness transformation!*

The final four weeks of your Anti Ageing Food and Fitness Plan really help you to shed those unwanted pounds and to increase your fitness level. You should also see a marked improvement in mood, energy, skin health, digestive function and fitness levels.

Your body will be reaping the rewards of more movement and those of an extended plant based diet.

You have been helping the body to naturally cleanse throughout the first eight weeks of your plan and enhancement of the digestive process continues in weeks 9 to 12.

This is the time to really focus on increasing your effort when doing the fitness part of the plan.

Whilst exercising, focus on what is often referred to as the mind muscle connection - when you are working out really try to be in the moment and notice and feel the different parts of your body that you are working out.

Make sure that you are getting adequate sleep during this period in particular.

Lack of sleep not only can make you look tired, it is also particularly taxing on the body and is detrimental to any anti ageing regime.

Anti ageing is really about wellness and to achieve optimum wellness you need to be rested.

You might like to consider taking some relaxing magnesium baths during this period or to try some guided meditations as these will help with better sleep.

There are some essential oils like lavender that may also assist.

A plant based diet that is colourful when combined with daily exercise, adequate hydration, relaxation and quality sleep delivers the best anti ageing results.

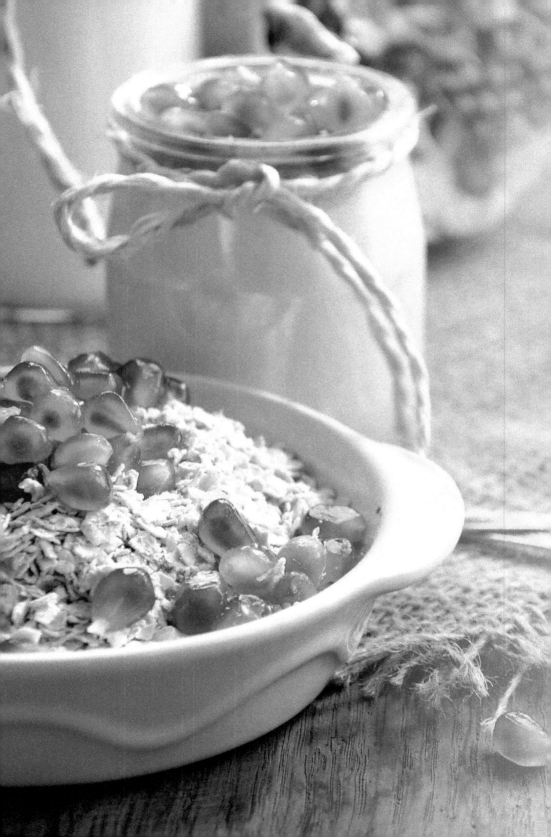

# Weeks
# 9 &11

## Renew

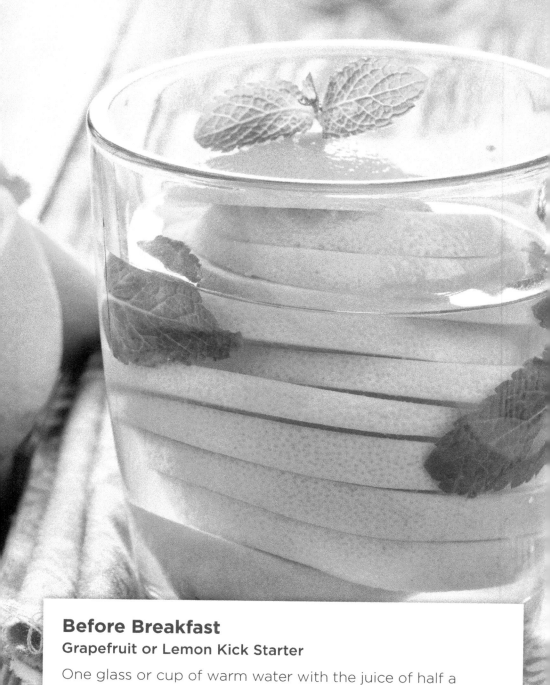

### Before Breakfast
#### Grapefruit or Lemon Kick Starter

One glass or cup of warm water with the juice of half a grapefruit or lemon in order to stimulate digestion and to help with fat metabolism.

Add a dash of cinnamon to stabilise blood sugar levels and reduce cravings whilst promoting a calm mood.

# Breakfast

### Spicy Baked Beans

Half a tin of organic low salt baked beans on 2 slices of wholemeal or rye toast.

Add some chilli or tabasco to the beans which act as thermogenic agents to speed up the metabolism and stimulate the digestion.

## OR

### Nut, Apple and Fruit Breakfast Bowl

Cut up 1 small apple and add a quarter of a cup of raw unsalted mixed nuts.

A few pieces of dried fruit such as dates, raisins or sultanas can also be added to help increase energy production.

Mix together in a bowl with a glass of unsweetened rice or almond milk – more energy and fibre from the dates and satiety from the nuts.

A handful of oats can be added to the mix to help promote fullness even more.

## OR

### Super Berry Smoothie

Blend 250mls of unsweetened rice or almond milk together with 1 small banana and half a cup of fresh or frozen berries.

1 scoop of plant based protein can be added to increase satiety as can a handful of almonds.

## AND

### Coffee / Tea or Herbal Tea

1 Cup of coffee, tea or herbal tea of choice – no added sugar or artificial sweeteners are to be used.

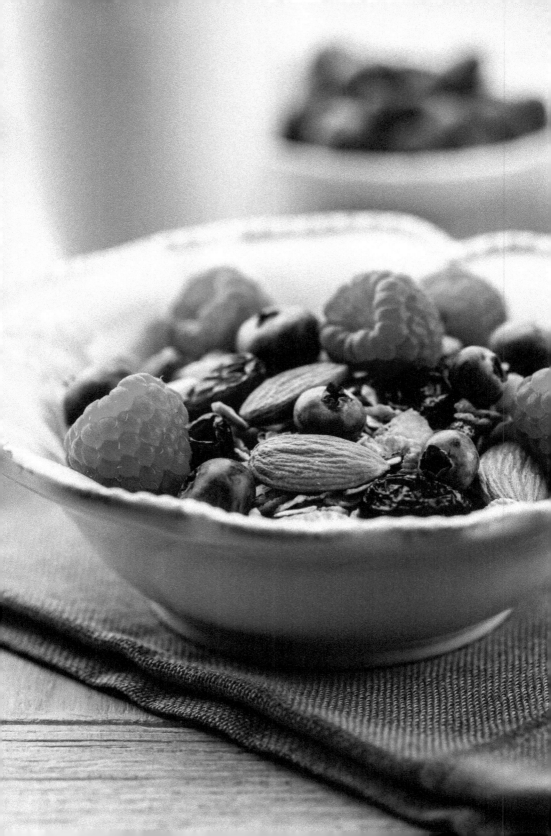

# Mid Morning

### Seasonal Fruit with Almonds and Seeds

Have a small bowl of seasonal fruit topped with 5 or 6 almonds.

This can be served with a few teaspoons of coconut yogurt.

The fruit and nuts are nutrient dense and help with both cognitive and immune function with the nuts providing protein to help with fullness.

### OR

### Apple and Pecan Snack

1 Apple with 6 – 8 pecans.

This snack combines pectin and protein to keep mid morning cravings at bay.

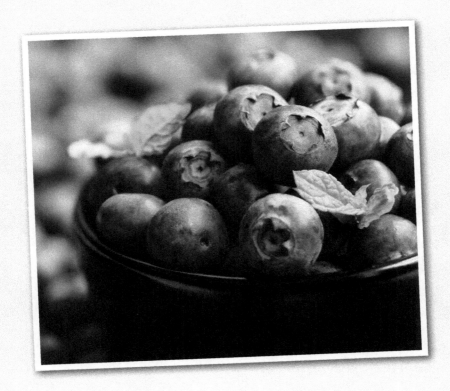

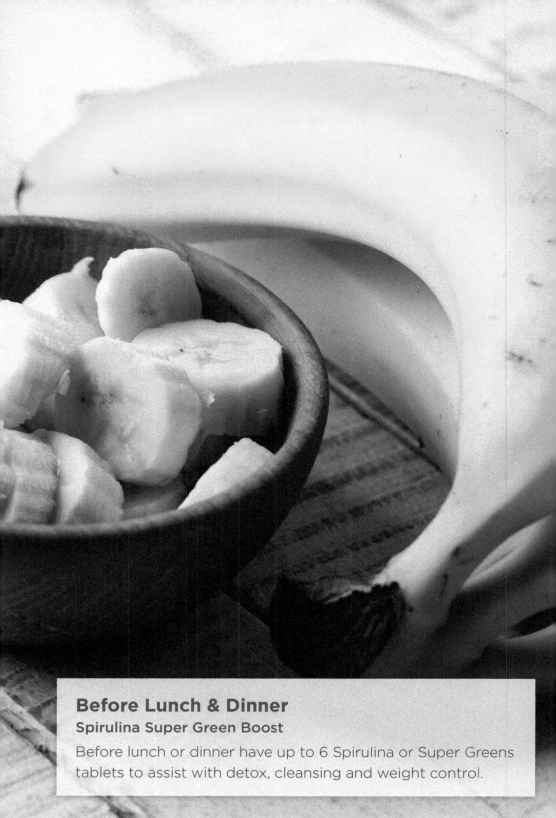

### Before Lunch & Dinner
#### Spirulina Super Green Boost

Before lunch or dinner have up to 6 Spirulina or Super Greens tablets to assist with detox, cleansing and weight control.

# Lunch

### Vegan Burger with Salad

Fry one vegan burger pattie in coconut oil and serve with a small avocado, onion and green leaf salad.

Add a handful of pine nuts.

Dress the salad in a little coconut oil with a drizzle of lemon juice and some craked black pepper.

### OR

### Rice Salad with Pine Nuts and Cashews

Add half a cup of any combination of steamed green vegetables to half a cup of brown rice.

Top with a handful of pine nuts and cashews to boost the protein content of this meal option.

Add spices of choice or a little tamari.

# Mid Afternoon

### Banana Delight

2 or 3 Dates or a glass of organic prune juice with 1 banana. If you're constipated it's harder to lose weight – the banana provides fibre and energy that will boost you both physically and mentally.

Have two teaspoons of mixed nuts and seeds if you want a higher protein content.

### Peppermint or Spearmint Tea

A cup of peppermint or spearmint tea with a little added honey to both calm and stimulate digestion.

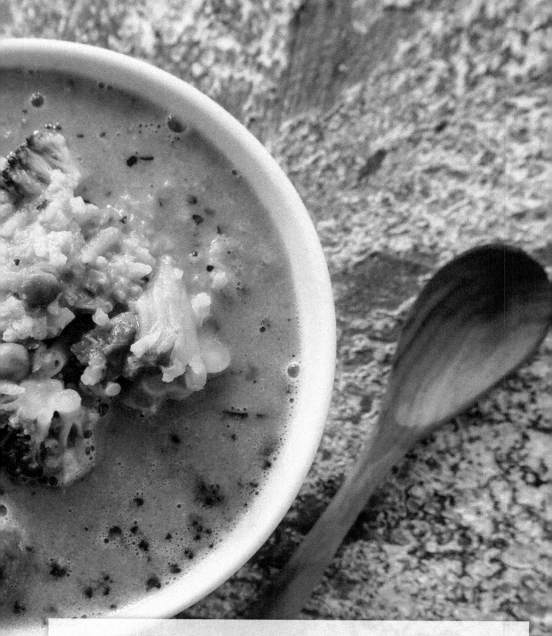

## Dinner

### Vegan Sausages with Mustard and Pine Nuts

Lightly fry two vegan sausages in cold pressed olive oil and serve with a cupful of leafy salad greens or steamed greens and a teaspoon or two of pine nuts.

Top with a mustard and chilli dressing.

**OR**

### Green Vegan Curry

• 1 tablespoon sesame oil • 1 tablespoon vegan green curry paste • 1 clove garlic • finely chopped • ¼ can coconut milk • 1 inch fresh ginger • cut in thick slices • cubed tofu pieces, 1 chilli cut in strips • 1 tablespoons tamari • handful of peas • three or four broccoli florets • quarter an onion and ¼ cup brown rice cooked

Stir fry all ingredients in a wok.

Stir in coconut milk.

Serve on brown rice when cooked.

**OR**

### Vegetable Stir Fry with Cashews

Lightly stir fry in cold pressed olive oil a vegetable medley of your choice.

Add 10 or 11 raw cashews and make sure you add spices to taste to stimulate digestive juices and speed up metabolism.

Serve with 3/4 cup of brown rice.
Use soy sauce, ginger, chilli and garlic.

**AND**

### Dandelion Tea

One cup of dandelion tea – the bitter qualities of this tea aid liver and gall bladder function making it good for weight loss, fluid retention, bloating and skin conditions.

## After Dinner

### Stewed Cinnamon Apples or Pears with Almonds

Slowly stew 1 apple or 1 pear and serve with a topping of cinnamon and half a teaspoon of almond slivers.

## Before Bed

### Sleepy Tea

1 cup of herbal tea such as chamomile, lemon balm or valerian.

# Exercises for **Weeks 9&11**

## Warm Up
### 1 Minute Cardio – Jump Ups

Start by having the feet fairly close together about shoulder width apart beginning with little jumps in the air.

After 10 seconds begin to jump up a bit higher from a squat position and start to also raise both knees in the air in front of you at the same time.

Try to make sure you land softly on your toes not your heels or on flat feet.

Increase intensity by jumping higher and faster bringing your knees up high.

Try to do for 1 minute.

## HIIT Circuit Weeks 9&11

Do each exercise in the circuit for 40 seconds intensely and then slowly for 20 seconds.

Each individual exercise within the circuit should be done for 1 minute.

You should rest for one minute after each circuit.

Try to complete the HIIT workouts three or four times a week.

For the LISS component of your fitness program you should aim to walk, swim, jog or cycle for 40 minutes twice a week

**Beginner** – complete once or twice

**Intermediate** – complete two or three times

**Advanced** – complete three or four times

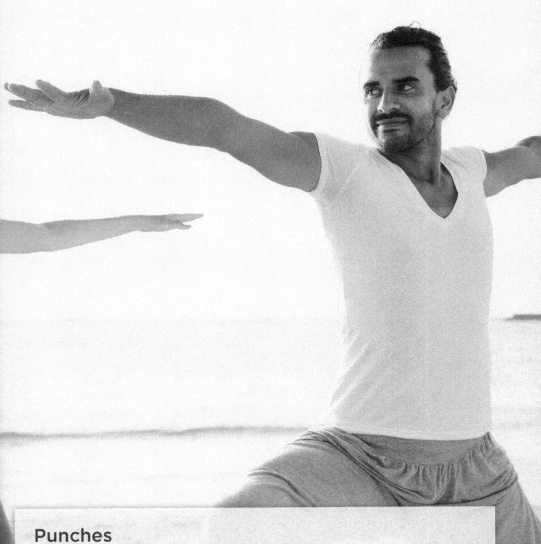

## Punches

Holding your hands up in front of your face punch forward in an alternating action.

Perform 10 forward punches and 10 hooks from side to side then 10 uppercuts.

Lunge Jumps

Start in a lunge position, then simply jump up in the air landing with your feet in the opposite positions.

Jump higher in the air to increase intensity.

## Superwoman

Start by lying down in a face down position. Stretch out your arms straight in front and stretch your legs straight behind.

Engage your core by drawing the belly button to the spine.

Take a breath in and as you exhale lift both the arms and legs (from the hips if possible) at the same time. Hold for a count of 2 and release back to your starting position.

Repeat.

## Abs Bicycle

Lay on your back with your lower legs in a tabletop position.

Slightly raise shoulders from floor with hands behind head.

Alternate moving your elbow towards your opposite knee in a fast motion, with your legs moving in a cycling action.

## Stretch & Relax
### Half Pigeon Pose

Start on all fours.

Bring your left knee forward and place it just behind and slightly to the left of your left wrist.
Place the lower leg at either a right angle (only for the most flexible) but probably at around 45 degrees toward the right inner thigh.

Stretch your right leg out behind you and fold your torso forwards and over your bent left leg – make sure to keep your hips balanced and don't over rotate. Hold for 1 min and repeat on the other side.

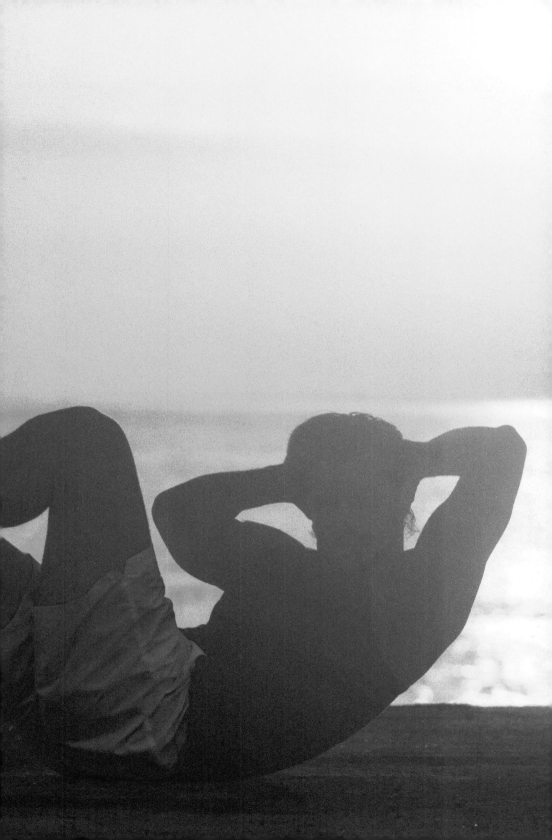

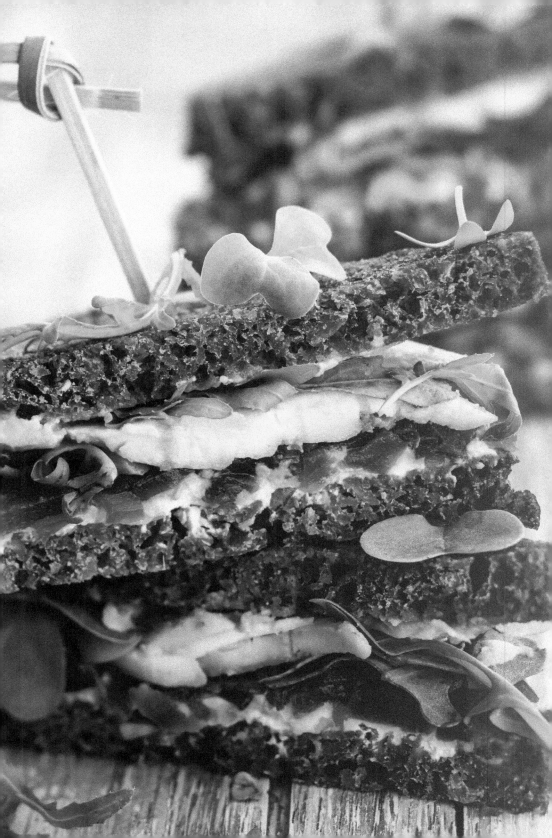

# Weeks
# 10 &12

## Renew

## Before Breakfast
### Lemon Grapefruit Blast

Have one glass or cup of warm filtered water with the juice of half a lemon and a quarter of a grapefruit.
Add a little cinnamon too.

# Breakfast

Do not eat breakfast for at least 12 to 14 hours after your dinner or dessert.

### Raspberry Smoothie

Blend 250mls of unsweetened rice • oat • coconut or almond milk with 1 small banana chopped • half a cup of raspberries and a handful of spinach or kale.

### OR

### Berry Bowl

1 cup of mixed berries – fresh or frozen – with a dollop of coconut or soya yoghurt.
The berries are a nutrient dense superfood that help keep your immune system strong whilst the yoghurt provides protein to help keep you full and focused.

### OR

### Chia Seed Porridge

- One cup of oats
- Rice milk or coconut milk
- One teaspoon of chia seeds and coconut flakes

Top with berries

### AND

### Green Tea

1 cup of green or matcha green tea to help burn and metabolise fat.

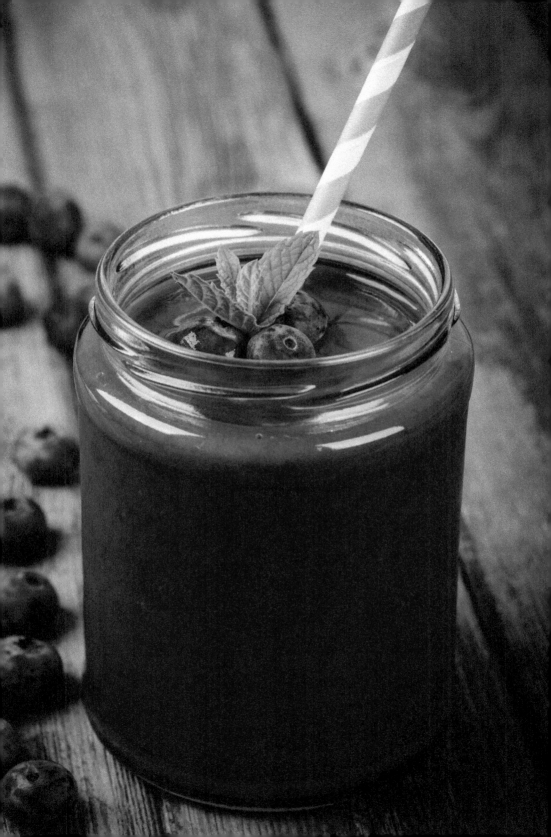

# Snack

### Prunes, Nuts and Seeds

3 or 4 prunes or a glass of organic prune juice if you prefer. Have together with 3 or 4 teaspoons of mixed nuts and seeds.

### Apple and Cashews

1 apple with 8 cashews will keep your sugar cravings at bay.

### AND

### Spearmint or Peppermint Tea

1 cup of herbal tea to keep digestive function at an optimal level.

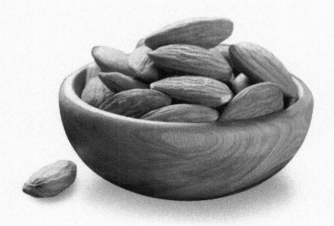

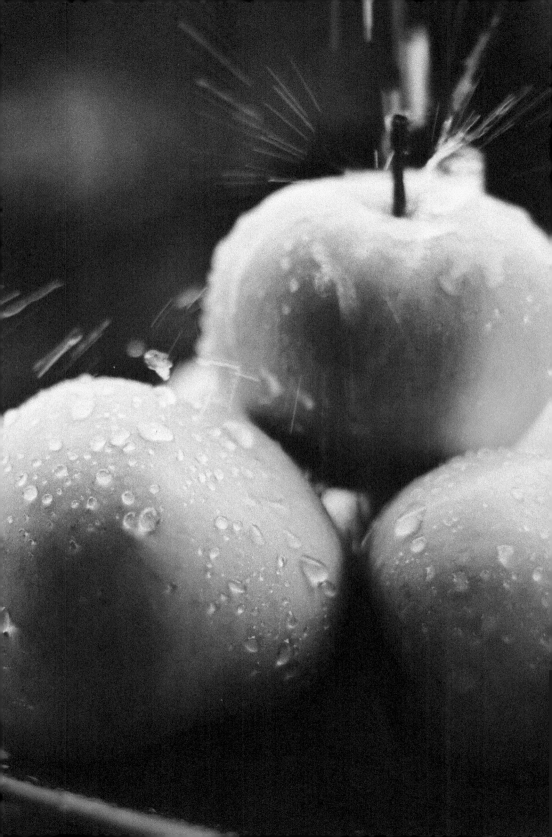

### Before Lunch & Dinner
#### Spirulina Super Green Boost

Before lunch and dinner you can take up to 6 Spirulina or Super Green tablets as they deliver high levels of chlorophyll to help reduce inflammation and assist with weight loss.

They may help to alkalise, cleanse and detox the system.

# Lunch

### Green Smoothie

• Blend 1 pear • 2 celery stalks • 1 inch slice of ginger • 2 cups of chard • ½ an avocado and 1 teaspoon of chia seeds with 200 mls of coconut water.

Add a pinch of chilli or cayenne for a thermogenic boost.

### OR

### Teriyaki Tofu Roll

• 1 tablespoon sesame oil • 4 medium sized sliced chestnut mushrooms • a pinch of salt • pepper to taste • 1 small vegan baguette or 2 slices of wholegrain bread • 2-3 teaspoons organic teriyaki sauce • five thin slices of tofu • 1 tablespoon tahini and small tomatoes to garnish

In a frying pan, heat oil over medium heat until hot.

Add mushrooms, salt and pepper, stir and cook/fry for about five-six minutes.

Add tofu slices and simmer for 5 minutes.

Cut small piece of roll in two halves.

Spread tahini on both halves.

Place tofu and mushrooms on one of the baguette halves and add teriyaki sauce on top.

Place the other half of the baguette on top.

**OR**

### Tempeh in Peanut Sauce with Brown Rice + Green Salad

• ½ pack of tempeh chopped into small squares • ¼ cup brown rice • 1 tbsp olive oil • ¼ cup chopped white onion • ¼ cup chopped green bell pepper • 1 tbsp peanut butter • 0.75 cup water • sea or rock salt as per taste • 1/8 cup crushed unsalted peanuts

Spices: ½ tsp of garlic • basil • oregano and soy sauce.

Fill your saucepan up to half and boil it.

Add tempeh pieces to it and let it cook for 5 minutes.

In the meanwhile heat olive oil in a nonstick pan and add the garlic, basil and oregano.

Thereafter sauté chopped onion.

Afterwards toss in chopped green bell pepper.

Let it cook for a few minutes.

In another small bowl combine peanut butter and soy sauce.

Whisk it smooth and then pour it in the nonstick pan when onion and bell pepper is properly cooked.

Sauté it for 2 minutes and add in the boiled and drained tempeh.

Immediately add 0.75 cup of water to it and salt as per your taste.

Mix it gently without crushing tempeh and let it cook on a low flame for 10-15 minutes.

Garnish with crushed peanuts and serve warm with brown rice.

Serve with Green Salad

## Mid Afternoon

### Raspberry Shot

- 1 lemon
- 0.15 litre still water
- 1 inch piece of fresh ginger root, peeled
- 8 -10 fresh raspberries
- Pinch of cayenne pepper

Peel ginger, and chop roughly. Add into blender. Squeeze lemon, and add water and blend.

### OR

### Mashed Avocado and Carrot or Celery Sticks

Half an avocado mashed served with 4 or 5 small carrots or celery sticks.

Have with a few olives.

### AND

### Dandelion Tea or Coffee

1 cup of dandelion tea to stimulate the liver and gall bladder and to assist with the digestive process.

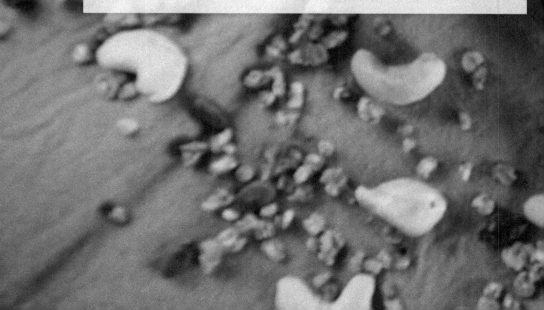

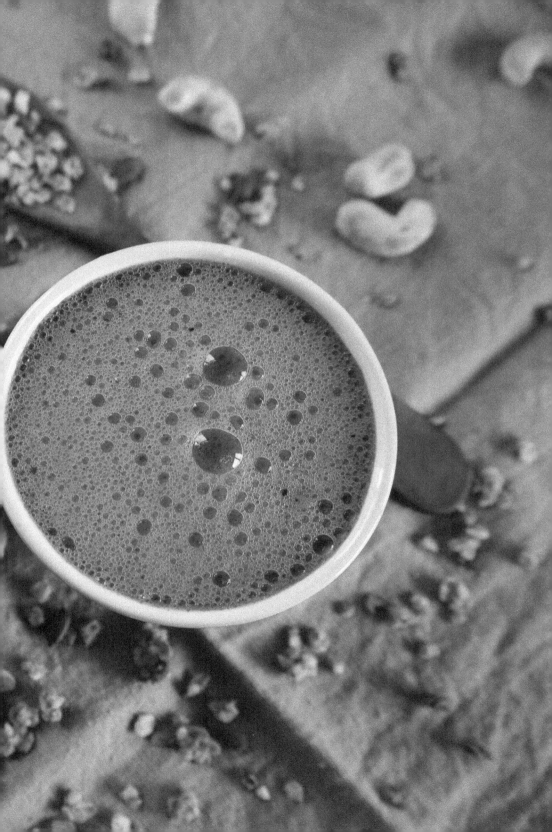

# Dinner

### Carrot and Coconut Soup

• 3 peeled and chopped carrots • ½ medium chopped onion • 2 cups vegetable stock • ½ can unsweetened coconut milk • sea salt • freshly ground black pepper and 2 tablespoons chilli sauce.

Blend all of the ingredients and add to a saucepan drizzled in about a tablespoon of cold pressed olive oil.

Cook for approx 20 minutes and top with a teaspoon of turmeric and a few slivers of almonds or some pine nuts.

## OR

### Chilli Roast Mediterranean Chick Pea Vegetables

• Any combination of 2 cups of vegetables such as red onion • courgette • peppers and tomatoes with a garlic • herb and chilli seasoning.

Add half a cup of chick peas.

Bake in a small lasagne dish with a drizzle of cold pressed olive oil.

Serve with olives and sun-dried tomatoes.

## OR

### Green Vegan Curry

• 1 tablespoons sesame oil • 1 tablespoon vegan green curry paste • 1 clove garlic • finely chopped • ¼ can coconut milk • 1 inch fresh ginger • cut in thick slices • cubed tofu pieces, 1 chilli cut in strips • 1 tablespoons tamari • handful of peas • three or four broccoli florets • quarter an onion and ¼ cup brown rice cooked

Stir fry all ingredients in a wok.

Stir in coconut milk.

Serve on brown rice when cooked.

## AND

### Anti Ageing Tea

1 cup of green or berry tea.

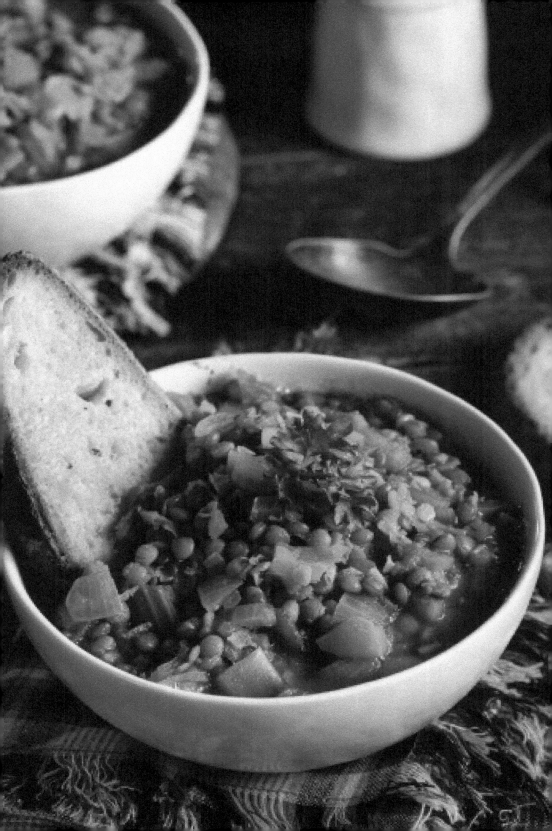

# Exercises for **Weeks 10&12**

## Warm Up
### 1 Minute Cardio – Star Cross Overs

Stand with your legs more than shoulder width apart with your arms out to the side and parallel to the ground.

Take your right hand and reach down toward your left foot bending forward as well.

Return to the star position and repeat on the other side. To increase the intensity increase the speed of motion, windmilling from side to side.

## HIIT Circuit Weeks 10&12

Do each exercise in the circuit for 40 seconds intensely and then slowly for 20 seconds.

Each individual exercise within the circuit should be done for 1 minute.

Rest for one minute after each circuit.

The HIIT circuit should be completed three to four times per week with a further two LISS exercise sessions on other days.

The LISS sessions can be 45 minutes of steady walking, slow jogging, swimming or cycling.

Beginner – complete once or twice

Intermediate – complete two or three times

Advanced – complete three or four times

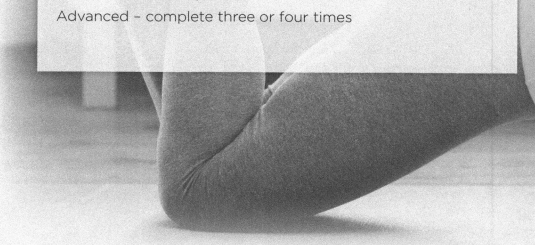

## Multi-Planar Jump Backs

The basic position here is a high Plank.

Begin by jumping the feet together towards the elbows to a crouch position then jump back to one side, i.e. about a 45 degree angle.

Keep jumping back and forth changing the direction to the other side.

Keep repeating all three positions, alternating sides.
To decrease the intensity you can walk the legs to/from the position so as to slow down the movement.

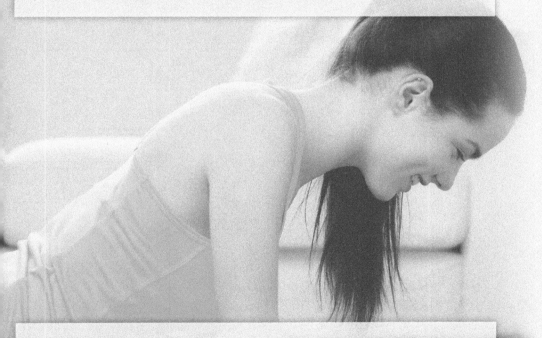

## Push Ups

**Beginners:** Start on your knees with your feet away from the floor. Keep your hips in line with your shoulders and knees. Keep the hips level and lower the torso toward the ground and push back to your starting position.

**Advanced:** Raise your knees from the floor and perform the movement on your toes.
Move your hands further apart to work the chest more and move them closer to work the triceps.

## Prisoner Squat & Kick

Holding your hands behind your head go down to a squat.

As you stand back up kick one leg forward on the way up. Repeat alternating legs.
Squat deeper to increase intensity.

## Abs – Leg Raise

Lay on your back with your legs straight up in the air with your soles facing the ceiling.

Raise the feet higher and lift the lower back from the floor, which exercises the lower abdominals.

Lower and repeat.

# Stretch & Relax

### Half King Fish Pose

This is a half spinal twist pose and a full body stretch.

Start by sitting up straight, with your legs out in front. Take the left foot and place it over the right knee.

Bring the right elbow around and place it on the outside of the left knee.

Place the left hand behind you – applying a little pressure on the left knee with the elbow.

Look over your left shoulder whilst feeling the full stretch.

To progress the pose bend the right leg round so that your foot is near your left glute.

Hold for at least 1 minute.
Reverse and repeat on the opposite side.

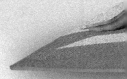

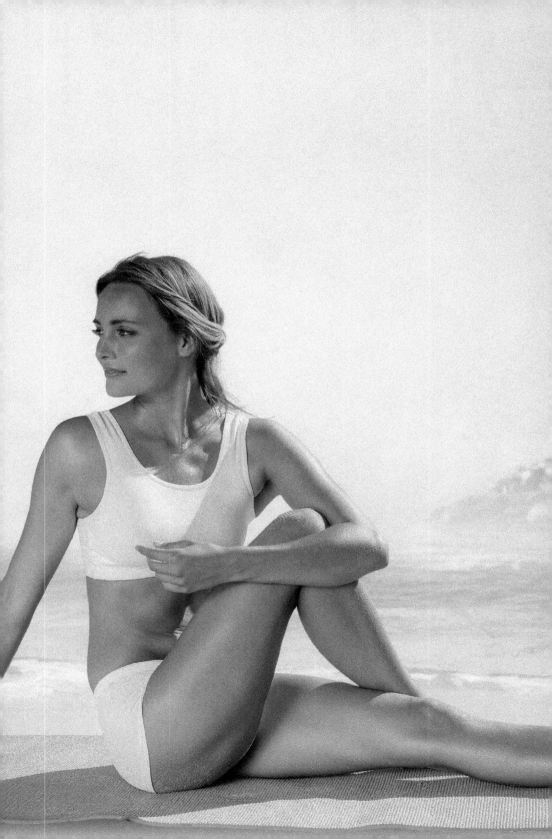

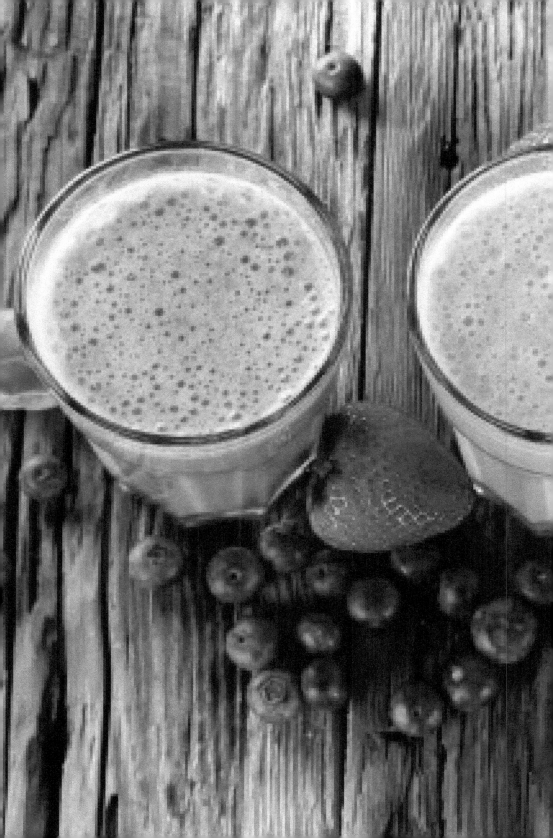

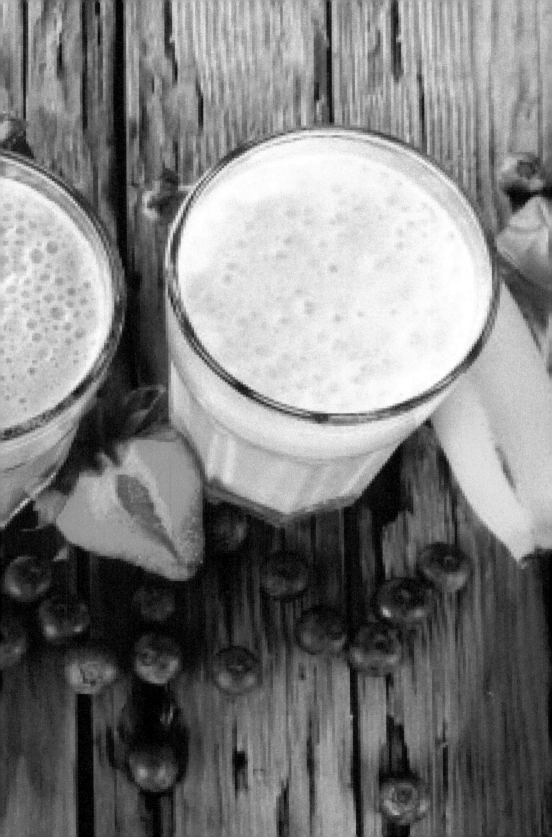

# Additional Breakfast Recipes
## by Daniela Fischer

### Quick 'n Easy Fig & Cashew Vanilla Protein Smoothie

- 3/4 cup raw cashews
- 1 cup rice milk
- 2-3 figs
- 1 scoop vanilla plant protein powder

Place all of the ingredients into your blender and blend on high until the desired consistency is reached.

Tip: Soak the cashews in water overnight as it makes the blending process smoother.

### Açai Bowl

- 1 pack frozen unsweetened açai berry pulp ¼ cup frozen blueberries
- ½ banana
- ½ cup rice milk

### Toppings:

- 1 tbsp chia seeds
- ¼ cup granola
- ¼ cup blueberries
- ½ banana – sliced
- 3 strawberries
- 1 tbsp goji berries
- Optional – drizzle of maple syrup

Mix the acai pulp, blueberries, banana and milk in blender until the desired con-sistency is reached
Pour the açai purée into a bowl and arrange the toppings.

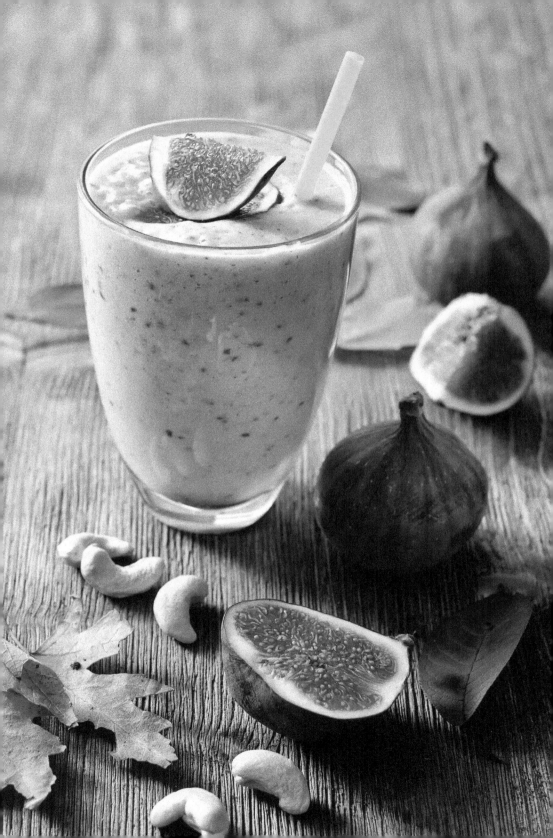

# Additional Lunch Recipes
## by Daniela Fischer

### Spinach, Quinoa and Roasted Chickpea Salad

- 1 ½ cups quinoa
- 1 can organic chickpeas
- 1 can organic corn
- 3 tablespoons extra-virgin olive oil 3/4 tsp salt
- Black pepper
- 2 thyme sprigs
- ½ tsp chilli powder
- 1 clove garlic, minced
- 1 tsp fresh lemon juice
- 4 cups fresh spinach
- 1 tbsp sliced shallot
- 1 tbsp cranberries

Add 1 ½ cups of uncooked quinoa to 3 cups of water. Boil in a medium saucepan.

Reduce heat to low – cover and simmer until tender and until most of the liquid has been absorbed for 15 to 20 minutes.

Heat oven to 200 degrees.

Toss the corn and chickpeas with 2 tablespoons of oil and season with ½ tsp salt and a dash of pepper.

Spread on a medium rimmed baking sheet and top with thyme sprigs.

Roast, tossing occasionally until golden-brown for 25-30 minutes.

Using a mortar and pestle, mash the garlic with a large pinch of salt until it forms a paste.

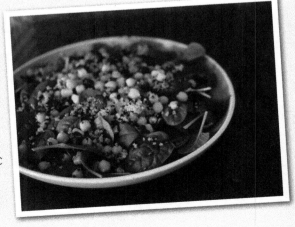

Add this to a small bowl and whisk in lemon juice and the remaining oil – season with salt and pepper.

In a large bowl combine the spinach, shallots, roasted corn & chickpeas and quinoa.

Toss with enough dressing to lightly coat vegetables and greens.

Add cranberries.

Serves 2

## Pumpkin Soup

- 300g pumpkin, peeled, chopped 1 potato chopped
- 1 carrot chopped
- 2 tablespoons olive oil
- 1 onion roughly chopped 1 garlic clove
- ¼ tsp ground nutmeg 3 tbsp coconut milk
- 1 ½ cups vegetable stock 1 tbsp pumpkin seeds

Heat the olive oil in large saucepan on a medium heat. Add the onion and cook for 3 minutes.

Add chopped garlic, pumpkin, carrot, potato and nutmeg, toss to coat.

Now add vegetable stock and 1 cup of water and boil.
Reduce heat to medium/low, cover and cook for 12-15 mins.
Cool for 20 min.
Transfer to a blender, mix until smooth.
Return the soup to pan and place over low heat.
Add coconut milk and season.
Top with pumpkin seeds.

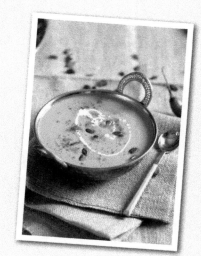

Serves 2 – large bowls.

# Additional Dinner Recipes
## by Daniela Fischer

### Baked Sweet Potato with Stuffed Rice, Chickpeas and Tofu

2 medium organic sweet potatoes ½ cup of
basmati rice
1 cup water
170g firm tofu – cubed

½ can chickpeas 1/8 tsp sea
salt 1/8 tsp cumin
¼ lime, juiced

1 onion
1 small cup of salsa

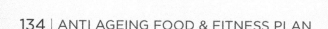

Preheat oven to 200 degrees C.

Put sweet potatoes in foil and bake for 40 – 50 minutes.

Rinse and drain ½ cup of rice.

Place in a saucepan; add double the amount of water and a pinch of salt.

Bring to the boil.
Lower the heat and cook on lowest heat for 15 min.

Remove the rice from heat and add the rinsed chickpeas and tofu.

Season with a dash of sea salt, pepper, 1/8 tsp cumin and 1 tbsp squeezed lemon.

Stir – adjust the seasoning as desired.

Add 1 tbsp of sesame oil and the chopped onion to a stir fry pan – transfer the rice mix to pan and heat for 5-10 minutes.

To serve split open baked potatoes and fill with the stir fry mix.

Serves 2

## Lentil & Squash Curry

1 cup butternut squash – cubed 1 cup
dried lentils
1 eggplant – cubed
½ cup water

½ cup coconut milk 2 tbsp garam
masala salt + pepper
1 tbsp coconut oil

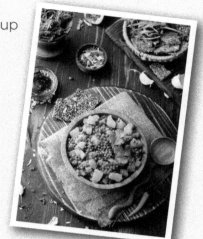

1 onion – sliced
1 garlic clove – minced
½ tsp ground turmeric
½ tsp ground coriander
¼ tsp cinnamon
¼ tsp chilli
1 handful coriander – chopped

Heat a little coconut oil and add the onion and garlic.
Fry gently for 4-6 minutes.
Add the squash, lentils and eggplant to the onions and stir
through.
Add coconut milk, water, garam masala and spices & simmer
on low heat for 30 minutes. Add more liquid if required.
Add the chopped coriander and cook for 5 more minutes on
a low heat.

Serves 2

# Fitness Tips
## by Ian Chapman

### Burn Fat Faster

So what effects how efficiently we burn fat and can we do it faster & for longer?

The best way to reach your goals faster and with better results is with HIIT.

This stands for High Intensity Interval Training.

Basically it's the principle of performing exercises at a higher intensity – going all out for a period of say 20- 40 seconds followed by a shorter period of either lower intensity or rest in between.

This style of training results in the burning of more calories in a shorter time than traditional continuous training.

Recent research shows that your body will actually burn more calories by doing HIIT and this will continue, even after you finish, for up to 2 hours.

This is known as the EPOC principle or Excess Post-Exercise Oxygen Consumption.

HIIT also creates muscle confusion – your body does not get the chance to get used to a particular exercise which delivers better fitness results.

You are less likely to get bored with this form of exercise and with most of us being time poor these days we can see better results in a shorter amount of time.

This is important as it means that you are more likely to stick to your routine and reach your goals.

Your body fat percentage will reduce and you will see improvements in blood pressure, general endurance and fitness levels too.

Muscle burns fat very efficiently so if you want to burn fat faster and increase your metabolism you need to work on increasing your lean muscle mass/tone.

This involves doing resistance exercises using both body weight and free weights.

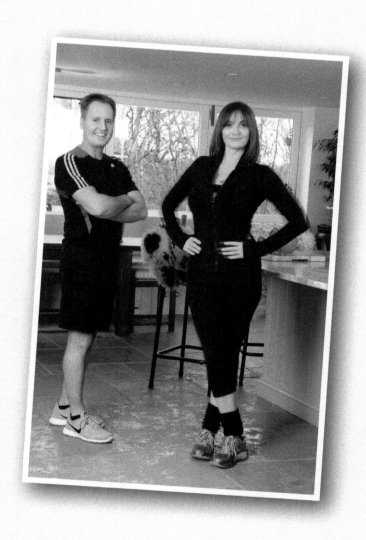

# Mindfulness Tips
by Ian Chapman

### Top Tips for Mindfulness

Chronic stress has negative effects on mental and physical health and can lead to an acceleration of the ageing process.

Mindfulness and Meditation can help to reverse some of the damage – the problem is that most people who try don't actually succeed or stick with it long enough to see the benefits.

With this in mind I have have put together a few tips that I think will help:

1. Read a book or two on the art of meditation or if you prefer get an instructional DVD, CD or App.

2. Invest in some relaxing music as this can really help take your mind off the stress of the day and create the right atmosphere to calm your mind.

3. Plan ahead – set aside time in the morning and evening to practice. It only needs be 5 minutes to start with and you can build from there.

4. Stretch before you begin and get comfortable – try to sit especially initially so you don't just fall asleep.

5. Choose the right place – be it your bedroom or a sun room etc. Just make sure you won't be disturbed. If unsure try an actual meditation class to get initial instruction. These are also available online so you can try one anytime.

6. Controlled breathing is the best way to begin – breathe in through the nose and pause – then breathe out through the mouth.
   This will help relax you and begin to clear the mind of chit chat and calm the nervous system too.

7. Be aware of your body.
   Imagine a white light slowly passing through the body – all the way down with the breath.
   Try to connect with your inner self.

8. Use meditation throughout the day.
   If you feel stressed, take a moment, breathe deep and move on from it.

9. Light a candle.
   Meditating with your eyes closed can be hard for a beginner.
   Use a candle as a focus point as this allows you to keep your attention stronger.

10. Make meditation be the first thing you do when you wake up – it will set the tone for the whole day.

11. Be grateful – give thanks for the good things in your life and try to maintain a positive outlook where possible.

You will no doubt go through a stage where you feel it simply isn't working.
This is when you really need to re-focus, re-read your books and talk to others who use this practice to help get you through.

Happy Mindfulness!

# Press Coverage

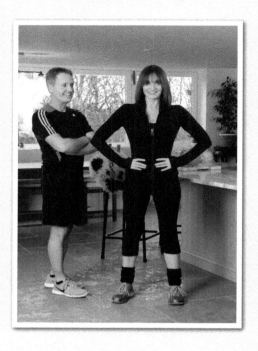

Actress Sarah Parish talks to Healthista Editor Anna Magee about how she lost a stone using The Anti- Ageing Plan from Healthista expert Rick Hay.

Despite having been a yo-yo dieter for years, it was only when she reached middle age that Sarah Parish really found a diet that worked for her – and it was anti-ageing too!

Sarah Parish was filming the first series of BBC Comedy W1A when she realised she had to do something about her body.

'I had a particularly tight skirt to wear and had already asked for Spanx but it just wouldn't do up,' she remembers.

'When they finally got it on me, I was bulging out of it and the bra they'd got me didn't fit because I'd put on so much weight since the last fitting.

The costume person said, 'It's okay, don't worry' and I remember thinking, 'Oh, don't pity me'.

That was February 2014 and a turning point for Parish.

'We'd been renovating a house during 2013, I was working a lot and then I lost my dad,' she remembers.

'Slightly depressed, I was drinking five cups of coffee a day and, always tired, I'd turn to sugar, chocolate, sweets, fizzy drinks, sandwiches, and packets of crisps eaten in the car.'

I'd gone from a size 10 to a 12 / 14 in six months and I was exhausted,' says Parish, who's starred in a string of top TV dramas including Monroe, Peak Practice, Cutting It and Mistresses.

'I knew if I kept going I'd have a middle aged figure – tummy spread, loose skin between the legs, cellulite – which also comes with the depression, the stress, the tiredness. I needed another way.'

Parish's five foot nine frame is now a small size 10. She's as stunning in real life as she looks on television, all cheekbones, long, slim legs and polished, dewy skin.

The whole picture is anything but middle-aged. So what's changed?

Parish is no stranger to diets and spent her 20s struggling to look a certain way. 'I fought against what I had rather than accepting it. As child, I wanted to be a dancer, was thin and boy-like.' Then at 16, puberty hit. 'I grew a pair of boobs and a bum and constantly covered myself up with baggy jumpers,' she remembers.

'I am athletic-looking with hips and boobs and knew I would never be willowy but it didn't stop me trying everything to change that.

Parish hired a personal trainer and started working out six days a week. 'We were doing High Intensity Interval Training [HIIT] with heavy weight training, lots of squats and dead lifts and also short four-minute bursts of cardio.' Though it didn't take long to get 'things into place again' there were still areas of stubborn fat that wouldn't shift.

Parish was working out but her diet had stayed the same. 'Some mornings I'd have avocado and poached egg, which is great but others I'd have five pieces of white toast then snack on crisps and chocolate.

This wasn't helping the dreaded tummy spread.

'I was complaining to a health-conscious friend about not being able to shift fat at the sides of my thighs, stomach and around my back and she said, 'There's someone I want you to meet.'

That's how Parish met Rick Hay, an Australian nutritional therapist who lectures in Sustainable Weight Management at London's College of Naturopathic Medicine.

Hay's plan emphasised focusing on a diet high in fruits, vegetables, plant proteins, vegetables juices and smoothies, designed to help her shift weight slowly, without counting calories. He got her off sugar and reduced her coffee to one cup a day ('by day five when the energy returns and your skin starts to look better it finally feels worth it,' she says).

Within eight weeks she'd dropped a dress size.

Hay's programme, explained in his new book The Anti Ageing Food and Fitness Plan is specifically designed to counter age-related weight gain by helping to increase metabolism.

The plan cuts out all refined sugar and processed carbohydrates and emphasised more protein from plant based sources such as pulses and beans.

It introduces 'thermogenic' (fat-burning) spices to recipes such as chilli, turmeric and cayenne pepper which studies have shown help increase metabolism after eating them.

The plan allows Parish, who enjoyed her wine before the diet, to have a glass of red a night.

To keep her sweet tooth satisfied, it features snacks such as smoothies made with naturally sweetened plant protein powders, berries, spinach and greens as well as healthy fats such as nuts and seeds to stop the energy dips that could lead to cravings for crisps or chocolate.

Rick taught her about the importance of building muscle with HIIT training.

One of the reason's Hay's plan also appealed was its anti- ageing element – so Parish didn't have to fall into the middle- age trap of choosing between a growing behind or a thin, but gaunt and ageing face.

'Rick taught me about the importance of building muscle with HIIT training and eating enough protein and nutrient rich foods to keep skin firm,' says Parish.

Within eight weeks she'd dropped a dress size.

The diet emphasises foods such as berries and greens like raw kale and spinach added to smoothies. These contain phytonutrients that have been associated with better skin health because of their antioxidant content, according to Hay. 'At first as I was detoxing my face went dull and a little flaky, but then I started to get more hydrated, drinking more water instead of coffee and my eyes were much brighter and my skin more plump. Now things spring back more than they used to.'

Still, Parish admits that especially in LA, the smaller girls tend to get the parts. 'Hollywood actresses look like little boys because the sad fact is that a tiny body and slightly big head tends to look better on camera,' says Parish. 'I have the opposite, a small head and a full, athletic figure so I don't compete with that. It's why I've always played evil queen types and character roles where you still need to be fit and have glowing skin but you don't need to be a certain size,' she says.

Parish then started filming a new TV drama called The Collection. 'It's all about the Dior New Look in fashion in Paris in the 1940s and the clothes are all cinched in waists and huge skirts, which I adore.' This time at the costume fitting she was delighted. 'Everything fitted! I had these French people going 'Oh, oui, belle,' about how nice everything looked and saying they had to pinch some of it in. That felt great.

My advice to anyone exercising who can't shift stubborn fat, is – change your diet if you want results.'

NB Sarah followed the original edition of 'The Anti Ageing Food and Fitness Plan' and now enjoys some of the recipes from this new plant based edition to stay in shape.

# Superfood Combinations

The term 'Superfood' refers to those foods that are especially rich in antioxidants, phytonutrients, vitamins, minerals, enzymes and amino acids. These nutrient dense foods can help to increase energy levels, boost immune function, improve digestion and help with weight management.

To further enhance results I recommend combining some of these nutritional powerhouses together:

## Energy
### Spirulina, Maca and Wheat Grass

Chlorophyll rich spirulina and wheatgrass contain high levels of magnesium which boosts energy production at a cellular level. When combined with the amino acid dense, South American superfood Maca, these three make a great pre-exercise option – a nutrient dense natural energy drink that's caffeine and sugar free. This blend will also help promote lean muscle mass after exercise which assists in fat metabolism and toning.

## Weight Loss
### Chia Seeds and Spirulina

Add a teaspoon of Chia Seeds and one of Spirulina to a smoothie in the morning to help kick start your metabolism. They are high in Omega 3 fatty acids so they will help with healthy hair, skin and nails and cognition.

They also help balance blood sugar which in turn, assists with optimum fat metabolism.

## Anti-Ageing
### Açai, Blueberry and Raspberries

This trio contains bioflavonoids, anthocyanidins and resveratrol – superbly powerful antioxidants that may help the body protect and repair itself. These produce positive benefits in terms of protecting the length of your 'telomeres' – little tips at the ends of your chromosomes that scientists have found shorten as the body ages. Longer healthy telomeres mean a longer healthy life.

## Digestion
### Barley Grass, Aloe Vera and Turmeric

To help reduce bloating and digestive problems add a half a teaspoon of barley grass and half a teaspoon of turmeric powder to a smoothie or juice and drink once or twice a day – add 5mls of antiviral, antimicrobial and antibacterial aloe vera juice to help soothe an upset tummy and to reduce flatulence. This combo has prebiotic qualities that will encourage the growth of gut friendly probiotics.

Turmeric contains a substance called curcumin which has been shown to work as a powerful anti-inflammatory.

## Detox
### Chlorophyll, Wheat Grass, Barley Grass and Spirulina

Cleanse and alkalise the system with these four super greens. You only need to add a quarter of a teaspoon of each to water or fresh juice to create a nutritional cocktail that will help to alkalise your system.

This is a good option if you are feeling really stressed or if you have been consuming too much much coffee, alcohol, sugar, dairy or meat.

The key to these superfoods is their deep green coloured pigments – these help to create an environment that is optimal for healthy digestion and elimination.

# Keep Your Body Young

Talk to any anti-ageing scientist right now and they'll mention telomeres. The longer yours are the better – and the slower you will age.

Telomeres are like protective bookends on the end of our chromosomes. Long healthy ones appear to be the key to protecting against age related illnesses and some would say they could be the key to slowing the ageing process itself.

You might have heard of the antioxidant resveratrol – rich quanitities are in deep red and purple foods such as blueberries and grapes. Resveratrol has been shown to both protect and lengthen telomeres.

I'm an advocate of a good glass of red every night with dinner but to get sufficient therapeutic amounts of resveratrol you'd have to drink hundreds of bottles which kind of negates the health benefits of the red wine.

There are other foods and nutrients that may assist in protecting telomeres and in the activation of telomerase.
Telomerase is an enzyme that keeps your telomeres in good shape and by having healthy lengthy telomeres, you will hopefully be protected from many age-related illnesses.

These foods not only protect telomeres but ongoing research is indicating that these nutrients that help to lengthen telomeres, increase energy and boost your immune system in general.

If you are looking to anti age the body try to consume more of these nutritional powerhouses.

## Antioxidants

Studies have shown that longer telomeres are associated with high antioxidant and polyphenol intake so think berries, wheatgrass, barley grass, chlorella, turmeric, hemp protein, astaxanthin, co-enzyme Q10, green tea or organic cacao.

## Folate

Lentils and spinach are perfect as they are high in folate, which promotes telomere health. Spinach makes a great addition to any juice or smoothie and lentils are a great source of protein and fibre to add to any soup.

## Magnesium

This mineral is believed to influence telomere length by helping with the integrity and repair of DNA so keep up your intake of dark leafy greens, nuts, seeds, avocados, bananas and figs.

## Leafy Green and Cruciferous Vegetables

Kale, spinach, watercress and other leafy greens are rich in immune boosting nutrients like vitamin C and beta-carotene with cruciferous vegetables that include broccoli, cauliflower, brussel sprouts and cabbage being natural sources of vhealth promoting glucosinolates and isothiocyanates.

These greens are also high in fibre to help with colon and gut health.

They help the body with it's natural detoxification pathways and promote healthy bowel transit times.

They are also rich in glutathione which is one potent free radical scavengers.

This antioxidant king may also offer protection to DNA structure.

## Onions and Garlic

Onions are garlic are both rich in glutathione also.

Garlic also helps to regulate blood sugar levels and may assist if metabolic syndrome is a problem.

They also contain diallyl disulfide which is very protective to the body.

## Orange or Yellow Coloured Fruit and Vegetables

The brightly coloured pigments found in orange and yellow plant foods are packed full of the super antioxidant carotenoids like alpha-carotene, beta-carotene, lutein and lycopene – all of which have immuno protective properties.

Falcarinol is a natural pesticide founds in carrots - it has promising anti cancer properties.

## Red Coloured Vegetables and Fruits

Tomatoes contain the antioxidant lycopene and diets that high in lycopene have been shown to help to reduce prostate cancer.

This seems to work well when served as tomato paste together with olive oil.

## Berries

Berries contain Gallic Acid to boost natural immune function and are rich in protective proanthocyanidins. They are also high in vitamins A and vitamin C. - both of which help with skin health.

They also have quercetin, zeaxanthin, lycopene and lutein as well as many other phytonutrients to help the body fight off pathogens. They are a true superfood in their own right.

A beetroot and berry juice provides an immune boosting enzyme rich juice that should be consumed daily at times when the system is compromised.

## Turmeric

The active ingredient is curcumin which is a key anti inflammatory agent. Turmeric may improve both heart health and cognition. It may also assist with improving circulation and helping to ease joint pain.

When used with black pepper, turmeric absorption is enhanced.

## Fermented and Probiotic Foods

These are key to good digestive health and help with nutrient absorption and probiotic levels.

Good gut function is integral to any healthy diet as without it key nutrients may be lost.

Foods like sauerkraut, tempeh and miso promote a healthy microbiome.

Research suggests that the microbiome may be one of the most important factors that determines overall good health and healthy immune function.

Apple cider vinegar also supports the health of your microbiome.

## Nuts and Seeds

Chia and Linseeds provide fibre for digestive system support together with omega-3 fatty acids to help decrease inflammation.

Nuts provide extra fibre, plant based protein and B vitamins for nervous system support also.

## Mushrooms

Medicinal mushrooms contain the immune booster 1,3-beta-glucan.

Varities like Reishi, Shiitake, Maitake and Cordyceps have been used traditionally for immuno modulation.

Modern research is now finding that both the polysaccharides and beta glucans found within the mushroom may indeed have these reported immuno modulating properties.

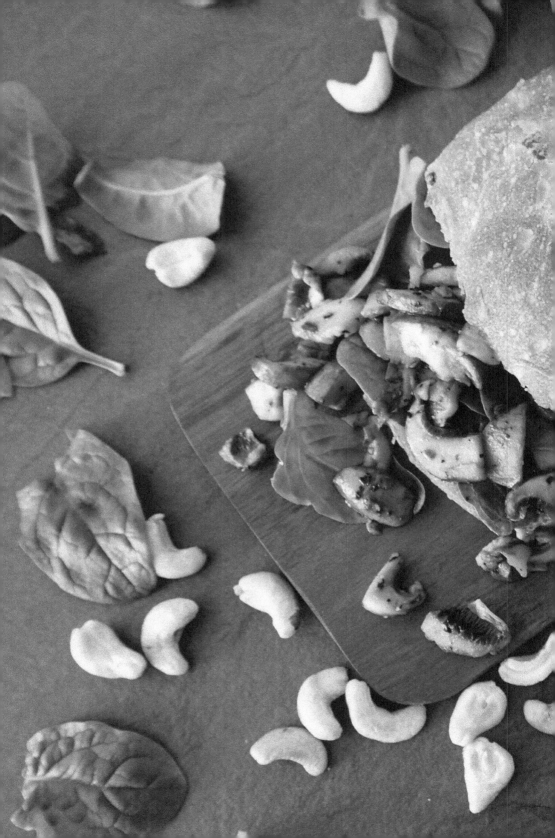

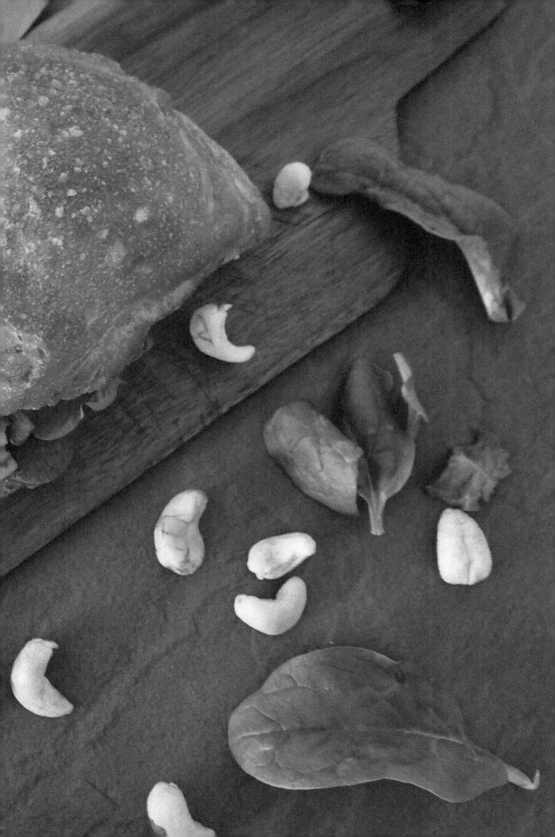

# What is a Superfood?

Superfoods – Do they exist and what are they?

Superfoods are foods that are nutrient dense and have strong antioxidant properties – a true superfood has a high Oxygen Radical Absorbance Capacity Score (ORAC). The higher the ORAC score the stronger the food's antioxidant ability.

This means that most true superfoods will have a positive effect on immune function.

Common colourful fruits and vegetables like raspberries, blackberries, beetroot, blueberries and spinach all fall into the superfood category.
They all have high ORAC scores and as a result are all good immune boosters in their own right – with beetroot powder or juice being the current standout in terms of enhancing sports performance.
When looking at everyday fruits and vegetables those that are brightly coloured are most likely to be considered a super food.

There is also lots of research currently being undertaken in order to identify the medicinal properties of common culinary herbs and spices.
The results for turmeric, cinnamon and oregano for example, are promising. turmeric has strong anti inflammatory properties whilst cinnamon is a great blood sugar regulator.
Oregano's anti microbial and anti bacterial properties also show promise.

I would even include some pulses in the superfood category – chickpeas, lentils and beans all are high in fibre and are rich in nutrients.
They are great foods to include into the diet to provide plant based protein – a diet that is high in plant based protein is generally the healthiest.

Foods that are high in fibre also assist with sustainable weight management, satiety and healthy digestive function.

Herbal teas such as liquorice, spearmint, raspberry, lemon balm and fennel and peppermint all have the properties of a true superfood.
These teas can assist with digestion, blood sugar regulation and immune function.

Like any true superfood they are powerful antioxidants that help the body in the fight against oxidative stress and free radical damage.

Teas can indeed be super, but herbal tinctures are like a turbo charged version of the tea.
Traditional medicine options such as globe artichoke, olive leaf, st john's wort, vervain and liquorice have been used successfully to treat a wide range of health conditions.

Even things like bitter salad leaves – chicory, endive and rocket – come under my superfood category. Their bitter quality stimulates liver and gall bladder function, which in turn, has a positive effect on digestion and fat metabolism.

I am a fan of the supergreen powders like spirulina, chlorella, wheat grass and barley grass to assist with alkalisation and cleansing.

I also recommend açai, boabab, lucuma, beetroot, watermelon, cherry and maca to help with energy production and sports performance.

Turmeric and olive leaf extract are two of my favourites when it comes to boosting immune function and fighting bacteria, viruses and microbes.

I think that adding algal oil to your diet is a good idea as it helps to improve cognition and mental performance.

Chia seeds are great to help with satiety and to increase the protein content of a smoothie – they are also high in essential fatty acids which help with healthy skin, hair and nails.

# Super Smoothies

Try some nourishing smoothies with a teaspoon or two of energising, alkalising, chlorophyll rich super greens or plant based protein powders like hemp, pea or rice.

Super smoothies tend to be high in magnesium and B vits to support the nervous system and also have good levels of energy producing iron and vitamin C.

Vitamin C not only helps with immune system function but has the added benefit of helping with collagen production so you may well find that skin appearance improves as well.

With their array of enzymes, phytonutrients and essential fatty acids these colourful smoothies make an excellent natural cleanser.

The addition of the super green powders also promote healthy digestive function and further contribute to skin, hair and nail health.

They can assist with regularity and help the body with its natural detox and cleansing processes.

Another bonus is that they also help to increase nutrient intake if you are not getting your five a day.

These colourful smoothies also help with energy production and may assist with weight management goals.

You may also find an improvement in skin, hair and nail health as essential fay acid levels are boosted.

A lift in mood and improvement in cognition may also be achieved.

Try one of these easy recipes for breakfast or lunch or as a healthy mid morning or mid afternoon healthy, nutrient dense snack option.

If you add in a serve of plant based protein to the smoothies you can use them as a meal replacement - they are packed full of amino acids and can help you to feel fuller for longer.

# Raspberry Cacao Treat

- 1 cup of Raspberries
- 1 teaspoon of Linseeds
- 1 teaspoon of Cayenne or Chilli
- 1 Date
- 1 teaspoon of Spirulina Powder
- 1 serving of plant based protein if desired
- Almond Milk

This super smoothie uses cayenne or chilli to help boost fat burning.

The pigments in the berries are great to boost immunity and they also provide energy.

The addition of Spirulina provides extra B vits and Iron to aid energy production.

# Blueberry Cacao Super Greens Smoothie

- 2 cups of blueberries
- 1 cup of spinach
- 1 teaspoon cacao
- one serve of plant based protein
- 200 mls hemp milk
- 1 teaspoon of Super Greens Powder

The blue pigments from the berries help to boost immunity. The cacao boosts free radical fighting antioxidants.

## Wheat Grass Sweet Green Smoothie

- one small avocado
- a handful of kale
- 200 mls coconut milk
- two prunes
- 1 teaspoon of Wheat Grass Powder

The avocado is a great source of protein and fibre to help reduce cravings.

The deep green pigments and added Wheat Grass help with detox and digestive function.

The prunes further increase fibre levels to assist with cleansing and satiety.

## Cleansing Chlorella Green Smoothie

- One banana
- Two figs
- Handful of english spinach
- 200 mls rice milk
- a handful of cashews
- 1 teaspoon of Chlorella Powder.

The potassium, iron, vitamin C and magnesium in this cleansing smoothie help with energy production.

The Chlorella powder helps with heavy metal detoxification

The cashews are high in protein which helps with muscle strength and endurance and they provide essential fatty acids for skin health.

## Barley Grass and Ginger Blast

- one beetroot
- handful of raspberries
- small piece of ginger
- 200 mls of coconut water
- 1 teaspoon of Barley Grass Powder

The Barley Grass provides extra energy boosting magnesium and iron.

The ginger soothes digestion and helps promote circulation.

The beetroot and berries stimulate nitric oxide to help deliver a natural burst of energy when you need it.

## Energy Super Smoothie

- 1 banana
- two dates, figs or prunes
- rice or almond milk
- a handful of cashews
- 1 serving of plant based protein

Blend the banana, two of the dates, prunes or figs together with 200 mls of rice or almond milk and a handful of cashews.

The potassium, iron, vitamin C and magnesium in this super smoothie help with energy production.

These nutrients are also essential to help fight tiredness and fatigue.

As this smoothie is rich in fibre it helps with weight management and to release energy slowly - so that you can train for longer.

The cashews are high in protein which helps with muscle strength and endurance and they provide essential fatty acids that help with cardio vascular health.

You might also like to try a superfood bowl - the are really just a thicker smoothie that you serve in small bowl:

## Rev Up Berry Superfood Bowl

- a small bowl
- a handful of english spinach
- a few blueberries and strawberries
- a banana
- 1 teaspoon of Chia seeds
- 100 mls of almond milk
- a dollop of coconut yogurt
- half of a sliced peeled kiwi fruit
- a few teaspoons of oats and granola if desired and some desiccated coconut.

Blend the almond milk, banana, spinach and pour into a small bowl.

Top with the blueberries, sliced kiwi fruit, strawberries, oats and granola

Top with a dollop of the coconut yogurt and some desiccated coconut.

It is an antioxidant powerhouse that will really help boost immunity and help with recovery and tiredness after exercise.

It's a mini multi vitamin/multi mineral in a bowl.

Good for brain function and mood too.

You can find my Sixty Second Smoothie videos online at healthista.com - there are thirty of them so there is lots of variety.

Here are 30 suggestions to get you started - notice that they are fruit and vegetable combos as these help to regulate blood sugar levels and consequently reduce cravings.

1. Raspberries, Blueberries, Chia Seeds, Linseeds, Cinnamon, Date, Coconut Yoghurt and Rice Milk
2. Avocado, Spinach, Dates, Prunes, Figs, Spinach and Coconut water
3. Pineapple, Banana, Apple and Coconut Milk
4. Banana, Date, Fig, Kale, Cashews and Almond Milk
5. Beetroot, Raspberry, Blackberry, Ginger and Coconut water
6. Raspberry, Cacao, Plant Based Yoghurt, Chia Seeds, Spinach and Almond milk
7. Mixed Berries, Oats, Seeds, Almonds, Spinach and Hemp Milk
8. Melon, Pear, Mango, Pineapple, Kale and Coconut Milk
9. Pineapple, Ginger , Celery and Coconut Water
10. Carrot, Kiwi and Coconut Water
11. Spinach, Apple, Pineapple and Rice Milk
12. Carrot, Apple, Ginger and Coconut Water/Milk
13. Watermelon, Cherry, Beetroot, Raspberries and Water
14. Cucumber, Lemon, Mint Leaves and Coconut Water
15. Melon, Apple, Grapes, Spinach or Kale and Water
16. Kiwi Fruit, Cantaloupe, Spinach, Blackberries and Coconut Milk
17. Strawberry and Tomato with Rice Milk
18. Banana, Fig, Date, Spinach and Hemp Milk
19. Pear, Kale, Kiwi, Cucumber and Coconut Milk
20. Orange, Apricot, Raspberry, Beetroot and Water
21. Pear, Pineapple, Mixed Salad leaves and Hemp Milk.
22. Passionfruit, Mango, Carrot and Coconut Milk.
23. Grapefruit, Orange and Coconut Milk
24. Prune, Pear, Spinach and Rice Milk
25. Peach, Nectarine, Carrot, Ginger and Water
26. Avocado, Pear, Melon, Spinach and Coconut water
27. Avocado, Strawberries, Coconut Yoghurt, Kale and Coconut Milk
28. Kale, Apple, Cucumber, Celery, Coconut Water, Pineapple and Coconut water
29. Peach, Melon, Pineapple, Mango, Kale, Coconut Yoghurt and Water
30. Blackberries, Blueberries, Banana, Avocado, Cashew Nuts and Rice Milk

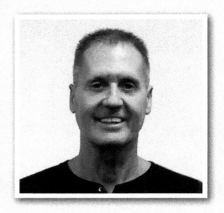

# Rick Hay

I am the Nutritional Director at Healthista so if you would like to check out more of my nutritional and fitness advice then go to www.healthista.com

You can also find a selection of my health videos there and on the Healthista You Tube Channel too.

More of my recipes, tips and a collection of my media coverage can also be found at: www.rickhay.co.uk

If you would like to follow me on social media I have two main Facebook pages: Anti Ageing Food & Fitness by Rick Hay and Rick Hay 'The Superfoodist'

I am also active on Twitter: @rickhayuk

My Instagram accounts are: rickhayuk & antiageingfoodandfitness

You also might like to take a look at my You Tube Channel: Rick Hay: Nutrition and Fitness.

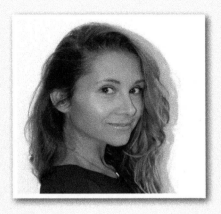

# Daniela Fischer

**Anti Ageing Food and Fitness Plan Recipe Creator and Photographer**

Daniela is a writer, recipe creator, yoga teacher and photographer who specialises in wellness and travel.

She qualified as a Hatha Yoga teacher at The Practice Bali and holds one to one classes and retreats.

She helps me to develop my nutritional plans, plant based recipes, herbal tonics and superfood formulations.

She divides divides her time between Bali, Los Angeles and London and will be working with me on my Plant Cure documentary that is being filmed in Australia.

Daniela is an advocate of plant based eating and is a firm believer in the healing power of nature.

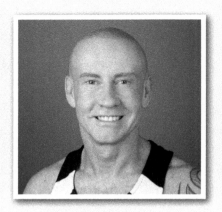

# Ian Chapman

**Anti Ageing Food & Fitness Plan Fitness Advisor**

Ian Chapman designed the fitness sections of 'The Anti Ageing Food and Fitness Plan' to deliver results fast.

He is a fully qualified, award winning Master Trainer, as well as a renowned Yoga and Pilates Teacher.

Ian has over 15 years experience in the Health and Fitness sector and has worked globally teaching the latest classes and holding educational seminars.
He has also worked internationally as the Fitness Director on a Luxury Cruise Liner.

He teaches in intimate 1 to 1 studio spaces and holds a variety of classes in large commercial gyms.
In addition, he visits and trains personal clients in corporate offices, writes his own fitness blog and appears in many fitness videos.

He regularly works on television in both the UK and Australia as a Guest Fitness Presenter.

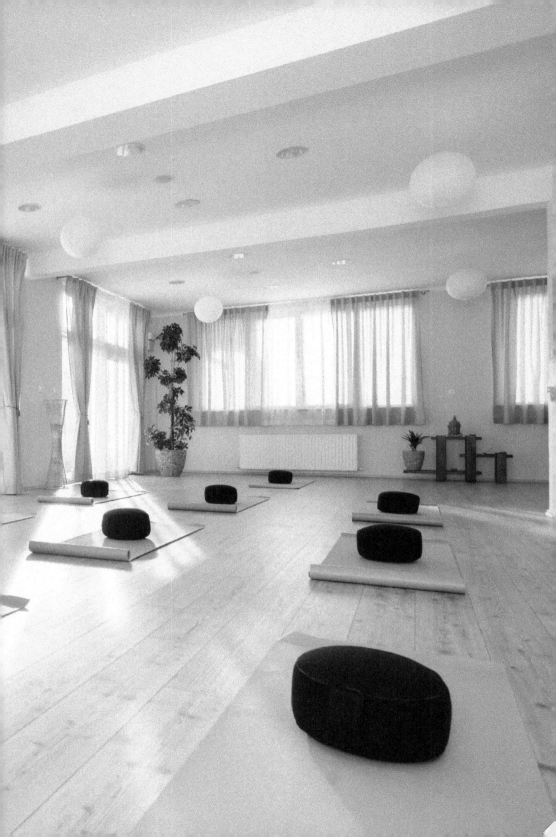